The Mindful Diet

Ruth Wolever, PhD, is a clinical health psychologist, the Director of Research at Duke Integrative Medicine, an advisor to the Duke Diet and Fitness Center, and an Associate Professor in the Department of Psychiatry & Behavioral Sciences at the Duke School of Medicine.

Beth Reardon, MS, RD, LDN, previously the Director of Integrative and Functional Nutrition at Duke Integrative Medicine and Senior Nutrition Advisor for Caring.com, currently has a private practice in the Boston area.

'*The Mindful Diet* provides an empowering program, gifting the reader with easy to implement tools to fully engage the mind in the fundamentally important decisions related to foods choices. This is extremely valuable information that will clearly enhance your resolve when it comes to eating right.'

    David Perlmutter, MD, FACN, number one bestselling author of *Grain Brain*

'This is not an "eat this, don't eat that" program; rather, it's an attack on the negative thoughts and patterns that lead to diet failure. Those who struggle with long-term weight issues may find this approach to be the answer they seek.'

Publishers Weekly

'*The Mindful Diet* gifts you with the tools needed to be mindful of every mouthful. Wolever and Reardon have transformed cutting edge science into a simple, doable blueprint for nourishing both mind and body. Reach for whole foods and redefine your relationship with foods as you let this elegant book guide you on your journey to optimal health and wellness.'

Pam Peeke MD, MPH, FACP, author of the bestsellers
The Hunger Fix, Body for Life for Women and *Fight Fat after Forty*

'*The Mindfu* with eating
and food. T don ground
the many su  cal research

and nutritional information. It illuminates the dimensions of mindful eating in a way that is easily approachable, yet can help break the cycle of overeating and over-dieting.'

Jean Kristeller, PhD, co-founder, The Center for Mindful Eating

'In *The Mindful Diet* you will learn which foods to emphasize in your diet and which are best avoided. But more importantly, you will learn how to transform your relationship to food from one of mindless eating to one of intention.'

Tieraona Low Dog, MD, author of *Healthy at Home* and *Life is Your Best Medicine*

'*The Mindful Diet* addresses the reason many people struggle with their weight – even though they know what they shouldn't eat, they still succumb to deeply ingrained habits, cravings, and distracted eating. With practical exercises and a sound eating plan, this fantastic, well-written book will teach you concrete strategies and skills for losing weight – for good!'

Cathy Wong, ND, CNS, author of *The Inside-Out Diet*

'If your goal is to stop starving and struggling with unrealistic diets and start making real, lasting, do-able changes to your eating habits, *The Mindful Diet* is an essential, must-read guide. *The Mindful Diet*, a sensible, practical, step-by-step guide based on decades of experience and research, is chock full of tips that map out a way to reprogram mindless eating habits right now!'

Dr Susan Albers, psychologist and bestselling author of *EatQ* and *Eating Mindfully*

'Wolever and Reardon's scientifically proven plan has effectively helped everyone from mindless eaters and yo-yo dieters to compulsive overeaters and binge eaters get a handle on their eating. Practice what they teach and you'll not only change your diet, you'll change your life!'

Jean Fain, author of *The Self-Compassion Diet*

The Mindful Diet

HOW TO TRANSFORM YOUR RELATIONSHIP
WITH FOOD FOR LASTING WEIGHT LOSS
AND VIBRANT HEALTH

Proven Strategies to Change Your Habits from
Duke Integrative Medicine

Ruth Quillian Wolever, PhD, and

Beth Reardon, MS, RD, LDN

with Tania Hannan

ATLANTIC BOOKS
London

First published in the United States in 2015 by Scribner,
an imprint of Simon & Schuster, Inc.

First published in Great Britain in 2015 by Atlantic Books,
an imprint of Atlantic Books Ltd.

This edition first published in Great Britain in 2016 by Atlantic Books

1 2 3 4 5 6 7 8 9

A CIP catalogue record for this book is available from the British Library.

E-book ISBN: 978-1-78239-650-5
Paperback ISBN: 978-1-78239-666-6

Printed in Great Britain by Clays Ltd, St Ives plc

For the gifted practitioners at Duke Integrative Medicine who opened my mind, the clients who opened my heart, and my family—near, far, and farther—who fill it with love. May you be happy, may you be healthy, may you be safe, and may you find joy along the way.

—B.R.

For my "Best Guys," Mark and Emma, who nourish me and sustain me, and for all the amazing clients who have generously shared their journeys with me.

—R.W.

For my mom, Evon Tefft, whose wisdom about food and health inspired a lifelong passion for both, and for my greatest joy, Stella.

—T.H.

Contents

Introduction

E very year, millions of Americans embark on the same quest: to lose weight and get healthy. We want more energy, we want to feel better about ourselves, and we want to live life more fully. And we know that at the core of all these changes is one roadblock: deeply ingrained eating habits. We know we need to make changes—the question is how.

There's no shortage of simple answers out there. But simple, quick-fix solutions—in the form of conventional diets—take people on roller coaster rides that do more harm than good, damaging both health and self-esteem.

At Duke Integrative Medicine, we've developed a revolutionary approach to managing weight that offers *real* answers and leads to sustainable change. As part of the Duke University Health System and as a national leader in integrative medicine, our clinic offers a new approach to health care. People come to Duke IM from all over the country to experience world-class medicine and complementary therapies—in a model that puts our clients at the center of their own care, and ultimately their own healing. Instead of focusing on isolated conditions and symptoms, we focus on "whole-person" health, looking at all the variables that can contribute to illness and to healing—including stress levels, nutrition and exercise, relationships, and even spirituality.

As a clinical health psychologist and as an integrative nutritionist, we've seen in our work with hundreds of clients that changing eating habits and losing weight isn't a simple equation of calories, pounds, and inches—and it's not about willpower. It's about our relationship with food, with our bodies, and with ourselves. *Authentic* change must come from within, and that's the guiding ethos of our work. The content? An innovative approach that combines proven behavior-change strategies with cutting-edge nutrition research to reprogram both the mind and the body, transforming eating habits from the inside out. Instead of skimming the surface, the way typical diets do, our programs tap into people's core values, the things that give them a sense of joy and satisfaction, and the goals they want to reach. And that's why they work. People in our programs change their eating habits, lose weight, and improve their health—not just for the short term, but over time. Such lasting change is possible because people experience a new commitment to their health and to their lives—and because the skills and wisdom they gain become part of who they are.

Using a foundation of mindfulness—a meditation-based approach demonstrated to help change behavior—we guide people to practice paying attention to what's happening in their minds and bodies, moment by moment. Because we live in a culture that discourages this self-awareness, gaining it is a revelation. People in our programs learn what true physical hunger feels like, and also what they're *really* hungry for. (Hint: It's not Cheez-Its.) Instead of the culturally ingrained all-or-nothing approach to eating—in which we restrict food, "fall off the wagon," beat ourselves up, and give up—people in our programs learn a nonjudgmental mindset in which every moment and every meal is new. Rather than treating their bodies as objects to be criticized and whipped into shape, they learn to treat them as worthy of care. And in place of the willpower myth that diets promote, they learn concrete skills to navigate our food-filled world and make better choices.

$\sim$

Laura is typical of the amazing people we've worked with who've shown us that lasting change is indeed possible—with the right intention, skills, motivation, and practice. Long overweight, she had tried commercial diets for years but always boomeranged back to her starting weight, blaming herself for lacking willpower. She came to our clinic for a consultation after her doctor advised her to go on medication—her blood-sugar and insulin levels, which had been creeping up for two years, had moved into the danger zone.

We didn't begin by asking Laura about her eating habits; we began by asking about her life. As with many of our clients, her life was very full—overflowing—and she liked it that way. She was an ob-gyn nurse, had two teenage daughters, and spent a lot of time helping her elderly mom. When she talked about her family and her work, there was warmth in her eyes, and it was obvious that she took pride in being the strong, caring center of her world—the person everyone leaned on. But her own health and well-being had been on the back burner for as long as she could remember. To keep up with her commitments, she had long ago settled into a pattern of eating "whatever's easiest"—the glazed cinnamon buns in the hospital cafeteria for breakfast, burritos and frozen pizzas for lunch and dinner, and diet soda as a quick pick-me-up during her long days. She had a nagging fear of what the road ahead would look like if she didn't change her habits—diabetes and heart disease—and when her doctor delivered the inevitable news, she was scared. As a nurse, she knew the devastating toll those conditions would take, not only on her but also on the people she loved. She wanted to change—*really* change—but she knew that dieting was not the answer.

While the diet industry corrals millions of women and men every year with seductive plans that promise to knock off pounds quickly and easily, most diets are counterproductive. Research shows that while people often lose weight through dieting in the short term, the vast majority of dieters regain the weight—and many keep gaining. In fact, dieting is a known *predictor* of weight gain. Dieting also takes people on a downward spiral emotionally, creating a cycle of success–relapse–weight gain that, when repeated, damages self-worth—which in turn undermines healthy habits.

The four-month program we designed for Laura was unlike any diet plan she'd ever tried. We didn't give her an eating plan and send her on her way. There were no weigh-ins, points, or calorie tracking. Instead,

Laura and the rest of the participants in her group took the first step toward genuine change—the practice of mindfulness. By learning a meditation practice and a set of related skills that helped them pay attention to what was happening within themselves—one that cultivated curiosity and compassion in place of judgment and self-criticism—Laura and her group were able to explore the root causes of their eating patterns: not *what* they ate, but *why*.

Laura realized, for the first time, that she had to look at her eating habits in the context of her whole life. Instead of perpetually focusing outward—on her job, on her family, on her to-do list, on a diet book, on the cinnamon rolls—she carved out time to slow down and focus on what was happening in her body and her mind. As it turned out, they had a lot to say. She practiced tuning in to her body's hunger and fullness signals, noticing her pattern of eating while stressed or exhausted, and paying attention to how different foods affected her energy levels. Instead of berating herself for making "bad" choices, she simply noticed them—and was amazed to find that this didn't amount to letting herself off the hook, but actually helped her to make *better* choices. She began to question the underlying thoughts that held her habits in place—including beliefs about herself ("weak-willed"), her weight ("never going to change"), and her life ("taking time for myself means letting other people down").

We've seen that our mindfulness-based programs help orient our clients to a new paradigm for eating and health—one that dismantles old patterns, provides new tools for making choices, and fosters deep, *internal* motivation. Armed with new skills and motivation, Laura felt her relationship to food shift. Instead of viewing food as simply fuel, or using it for comfort, she began to realize how deeply her choices impacted her health, for better or worse, and changed her eating accordingly. And rather than focusing on the *quantity* of food she ate—calories and portions—she began focusing on the *quality*.

Our nutritionists teach people what different foods and beverages do in the body on a biochemical level—and how everything we consume moves us toward health or illness. As it turns out, eating for a balanced weight and eating for overall health are one and the same. If your body's cells could talk, we like to say, they'd make their menu choices loud and clear: a whole-foods, plant-based diet—the template of global cuisines celebrated for their health benefits. Such an eating plan is the body's best defense against obesity *and* the chronic illnesses that we're susceptible to as a result of our genetics and our environment.

Laura started keeping her values and her inner wisdom at the forefront of her mind and using those internal resources as guides when she made decisions about eating and exercise. She started eating more vegetables, whole grains, and fish—which had the effect of "crowding out" her intake of processed foods, soda, and sweets. Once she stopped eating those former standbys, she began to lose her taste for them. Instead of grabbing whatever was easiest, she made time to plan, shop for, and cook meals—and realized that even when she had to eat on the run, she had choices. She also started choosing to walk on her lunch break, instead of working through it; she'd never felt like she had the time before, but now she made the time.

Laura stuck with these changes and her mindfulness practices long past the program's ending—not because someone was telling her to, but because she could feel the difference it was making in her body and in her life. The changes became her new habits—who she was and how she lived. Just as steadily as they had risen, her blood-sugar and insulin levels started to drop, along with her weight, and she was able to stop taking medication. In a year and a half, she had lost 25 pounds, and her blood-sugar and insulin levels had normalized.

Our Stories: Ruth Wolever, Ph.D.

As a clinical health psychologist and Duke Integrative Medicine's director of research, I have been working with people individually and in groups on changing their habits for more than twenty years—and studying what works best. It's a given in my field that changing deeply ingrained habits such as overeating requires looking at our internal landscapes—thoughts, beliefs, and emotions—as opposed to following an "external" approach like dieting. But the question is, how do we shift that internal landscape? While traditional cognitive behavioral therapy—which focuses on changing thoughts in order to change behavior—is enormously helpful, I've found that it doesn't go far enough for many people.

My doctoral research on mind-body health, the burgeoning research on the power of mindfulness meditation, and my own experience with meditation led me to begin incorporating mindfulness into my work with individual clients and in groups—and I was amazed at how powerful it was in helping people change their eating patterns. It takes work to recognize what drives our habits, but that's what people in our programs figure out: what really drives their eating habits, what their minds make up, what they choose to believe, and how to align their behavior with what they most care about.

Across my twenty years of practice, I have had the incredible opportunity to work closely with, and learn from, hundreds of remarkable clients. I share their aggravation with a society that presents a very mixed message: eat, consume, buy more—but somehow get yourself to look like an Athleta model. One of the universal lessons I see in my work is that when we expend our energy looking outward and trying to keep up with life, it's easy to forget that we are *creating* that very life—that we actually have a great deal of power in shaping our worlds. Forgetting our internal world—not paying attention to our deepest selves—is a byproduct of the cultural messages of immediate gratification and "quick fixes" that surround us. There is no quick fix for the complex eating patterns we've developed over years, but there are ways to "fix them well." What people need are the tools to get in touch with their own deep wisdom—and that's what our programs offer.

Our Stories: Beth Reardon, M.S., R.D., L.D.N.

The *science* of what I do as an integrative nutritionist is rooted in nutritional biochemistry and functional medicine. The *heart* of what I do is to help people get in touch with who they are as they're moving through this world—physically, emotionally, and spiritually—and how changing their relationship with food can help them achieve their goals.

Shifting that relationship is often not a linear path. When I came to Duke Integrative Medicine in 2007, I began to understand why not all my clients heeded my advice and "got better." I had believed that if people knew the right information—the biochemistry of food, the health statistics—they would change. But the integrative model helped me to understand that changing behavior is rarely about the information; it's about figuring out what's keeping us stuck and unable to make shifts in our lives. Often it has to do with our family food histories. In one case, a client had trouble giving up her nightly slice of pie after dinner. As it turned out, the pie was part of a ritual she had shared with her father. How could I ask her to change that? What I *could* do, I realized, was to help her see that there were other ways to nurture memories of that loving relationship—while guiding her in implementing an eating plan that supported her health and helped her achieve her goals.

Clients I see who've been overweight for a long time or have a serious health condition are sometimes fatalistic. But everyone can improve their health by nourishing themselves well. Food affects our very DNA, and every bite matters—it really does. I've worked with so many clients who've changed their health trajectories by changing their habits. It takes a committed effort because of the food culture we're living in and our entrenched patterns. But eating well is simpler than most people think. In fact, in general, the simpler we eat, the better. It begins with setting the intention to choose foods that *matter*—foods that are worthy of us.

∼

In scores of patients who've gone through our programs, we've seen that the negative spiral of eating, weight, and health can become a positive one. And our research supports this. We've tested our mindfulness-based approach in several NIH-funded studies and a large industry study. Results show that our programs helped people decrease overeating, lose weight gradually, and maintain that weight loss over time. The most remarkable part is that participants reported losing weight and maintaining weight loss *without a struggle*. Mindfulness training has also been shown to improve metabolism irrespective of weight loss; in one study, two groups received the same eating advice, but one of the groups received training in mindfulness. Those who practiced mindfulness digested and absorbed food—especially carbohydrates—more efficiently. They also reported being less likely to overeat sweets and high-fat foods—and being satisfied with far smaller portions than they had previously eaten. These results underscore that our mindfulness-based approach can help people connect with the innate feedback systems that naturally regulate eating and weight—in other words, make authentic change from within.

People who follow our program start to care deeply about what they put in their bodies, often for the first time in their lives. We've found that when people start nourishing themselves with the right foods, even after decades of not doing so, their very taste buds change. A ripe nectarine, for instance, becomes the perfect dessert. By reprogramming their minds, they're able to reprogram their bodies.

~

For the first time, we are offering our approach in book form so that people everywhere can reap the benefits. *The Mindful Diet,* an antidote to both unhealthy eating patterns and the diet roller coaster, takes you through a step-by-step program that will help you transform your relationship with food, lose excess weight if you need to (and keep it off), and eat in a way that deeply supports your body's health—while keeping your taste buds happy and feeding your spirit.

The Mindful Diet is divided into three parts, with concepts, skills, and tools that build on one another. It's best to work through the chapters in sequence instead of skipping around. Because you'll be learning new skills and implementing changes throughout, spend about a week on each chapter—and take more time if you need it. Slow, incremental progress is much more effective and sustainable than sudden, wholesale overhauls.

In **Part I, Setting the Stage for Change,** we'll shine a light on three powerful factors that make unhealthy eating almost automatic: our food culture, the lack of balance in our lives, and the influence of the diet industry. You'll learn about how both food companies and our overscheduled lives encourage eating for the wrong reasons and why getting in touch with your values will help you eat for the right ones. You'll also find out why the diet mentality that permeates our culture is built on false promises that set people up to fail—and how to break free from it. In **Part II, Building Your Foundation,** you'll begin a meditation practice and learn how to apply mindful awareness to your eating habits. You'll learn the difference between true hunger and its many imposters, discover your unique "stress profile" and how it affects your eating habits, and begin to stop judging your body and start *inhabiting* it. The skills you'll develop in this section—your mindfulness toolkit—will work to dismantle unhealthy patterns and build a solid foundation for healthy, sustainable habits.

With your foundation in place, you'll be ready to build a way of eating that truly supports your health. In **Part III, Eating for Total Health,** you will learn how different foods affect your body on the cellular level, either encouraging or discouraging conditions like obesity, insulin resistance, and diabetes—and how to crowd out unhealthy choices with simple, delicious, health-promoting food. We'll guide you in getting a handle on your portions and reorganizing your kitchen and your life for healthy eating—with help from shopping lists, mix-and-match meal charts, dining-out advice, and healthy cooking techniques.

What You'll Need to Start

- *A journal.* The program involves written exercises and reflection, so you'll need a notebook or journal. It doesn't have to be fancy or large—in fact, you'll want something that you can easily carry with you, but with ample space to write. A 5-by-7-inch notebook would work well.

- *Time.* The exercises and meditations in the program will require fifteen to thirty minutes per day. To help ensure that you'll follow through, set aside a specific time, in the same way you'd do for an appointment.

- *Support.* Round up a few people close to you, family or friends, and tell them you're embarking on a program to change the way you live and would like their support.

~

The Mindful Diet will help you reconnect (or connect for the first time)—to your food, and to your body and mind. That might sound like a tall order, but all of those factors are inextricably linked, whether they're functioning in unhealthy ways or in harmony. The payoff? Long-term changes in habits that lead to better balance—on your plate, for your health, and in your life.

Once you start to reap the rewards of listening to your body and nourishing it, healthy eating will no longer be something you *should* do; it will be something you *want* to do, and can do naturally, because it feels good and because you feel good—about yourself, and about what, how, and why you're eating. And that's powerful medicine.

PART I

Setting the Stage
for Change

CHAPTER 1

Why We Overeat

"When walking, walk. When eating, eat."

—Zen proverb

Picture this: A woman sits down at a table to eat, closing her eyes for a moment to take a long, deep breath. She's hungry, but not stomach-growling, light-headed famished. On her plate are sautéed Swiss chard, roasted winter squash, wild salmon with ginger, and a salad. She takes a moment to consider all it took to create this moment, from the farmers who grew the vegetables to herself for making time to shop for the groceries and thoughtfully prepare the meal, and feels grateful. She eats slowly, savoring the earthy flavor of the greens, the salad's tangy crunch, and the creamy sweetness of the squash. She pauses to put her fork down between bites, sips a mug of green tea, and checks in with her body. When she senses that she's had enough food—feeling satisfied but nowhere near stuffed—she stops.

That's lovely, you might be thinking, *but that's not real life.* Real-life eating is often the polar opposite of the scene above.

In real life, you're trying to get a frozen pizza in the oven with one child pulling at your leg and the other needing help with homework.

Or you're alone, and who wants to go to the trouble of slicing vegetables when ordering Chinese takeout is so easy? In real life, "breakfast" was coffee on the way to work, the staff meeting starts in five minutes, and the bag of Doritos on your desk is looking good. In real life, you aren't hungry, but not eating your mother-in-law's chicken potpie feels rude, so you stuff it down. In real life, talking to your critical older sister triggers a Pavlovian response for dulce de leche ice cream. In real life, you blew your diet last night at your best friend's birthday bash, so all bets are off, and the fluorescent Taco Bell sign up the road is beckoning like a siren. In real life, you ordered a veggie sub for lunch and it's a *foot long*, and while you didn't ask for potato chips, here they are. In real life, chocolate is the most reliable, consistent pleasure you know. In real life, every diet you've tried has left you feeling two things: hungry and unhappy.

You can probably think of a dozen other examples of how real life seems to undermine your desire to be a healthy eater. What seems on one level like a simple, straightforward act—nourishing our bodies—is often complicated by forces that feel beyond our control.

The New Status Quo: Mindless, Automatic Eating

It's normal to eat too much, eat too quickly, eat for comfort, or choose unhealthy food on occasion. But for increasing numbers of people, these habits are not the exception; they're the norm. There are many reasons this is so, which we'll explore, but the underlying reality is that we often engage in the incredibly important act of nourishing our bodies without fully recognizing what we're doing, and this has serious consequences. Consider the common habit of eating while doing other things—whether that's driving, checking email, walking through the grocery store, or watching TV. Research shows that when people eat while they're distracted or multitasking, they eat faster, eat a bigger portion, don't remember what they consumed, feel significantly less full, and continue to eat more *throughout the day*.

In this book, we refer to unconscious eating—driven by habit and convenience rather than our wisest selves—as mindless eating. Does that mean you sleepwalk to the kitchen and wake up with the taste of French fries or chocolate cake in your mouth, remembering nothing? No, though for some people, eating feels like that. For most of us, though, eating is often what psychologists call an automatic behavior, akin to walking or driving (once we've learned those skills). Automatic behaviors are activities that have become so second nature to us that we do them on autopilot, without paying full attention and often while doing other things.

Automatic behaviors aren't unhealthy by definition. If you've watched a baby learn how to walk, you know that the task consumes all of her attention. But eventually it becomes automatic, and that frees her up to do other things while walking. That's why as adults we can walk and talk, or walk and think, or walk and listen to music. The autopilot nature of eating, however, tends to get us into trouble when our environment is rife with unhealthy eating options and distractions. For many of us, it takes a great deal of attention and effort to make healthy choices. Autopilot eating also makes it too easy to eat for reasons other than hunger, and to not even notice we're doing so.

Very often it's a combination of limited time, stress, opportunity, and our own emotional landscape that prompts us to take that first bite and keep eating. Our culture, along with the nature of our brains, has created a perfect storm that encourages us to automatically eat, overeat, or eat unhealthy food.

Mindless-Eating Checklist

Mindless eating comes in many forms. You may not have a clear sense of your eating behavior at this point, and that's okay. This checklist can help you begin to tune in to your own eating patterns and habits.

I do the following . . .	rarely	some-times	often
Eat until I'm uncomfortably full	❑	❑	❑
Eat until I'm stuffed	❑	❑	❑
Eat very quickly, consuming a meal in less than ten minutes	❑	❑	❑

I do the following . . .	rarely	some-times	often
Eat while standing up or walking	❑	❑	❑
Eat while driving	❑	❑	❑
Eat when I'm not hungry	❑	❑	❑
Eat because food "is there"	❑	❑	❑
Eat while watching television	❑	❑	❑
Eat in front of the computer	❑	❑	❑
Wait until I'm extremely hungry to eat	❑	❑	❑
Eat in response to stress or anxiety	❑	❑	❑
Eat in response to depression, loneliness, or sadness	❑	❑	❑
Eat in response to anger or frustration	❑	❑	❑
Eat in response to boredom	❑	❑	❑
Eat fast food and convenience food because I haven't planned	❑	❑	❑
Eat just because others are eating	❑	❑	❑
Eat because the clock says it's time to eat	❑	❑	❑
Know I'm finished when the plate or package is empty	❑	❑	❑

Take a look at any areas that you answered as "often" and "sometimes," and pay attention to these habits as you go through the program. It's normal to do all of these once in a while, but they undermine your health when done with any regularity. Shifting to "rarely" for all the areas above is ideal—but getting there is a process. You'll be learning more about all of these patterns throughout the book.

Our Food Culture: Fast, Cheap, and Out of Control

We all know the cliché that we're products of our environment, and numerous studies over the past decade have shown how true this is for eating in particular. Research shows that human beings tend to eat food we see that's within reach, *regardless of our level of hunger or how the food truly tastes.*

And oh, the food we see! Our surroundings are filled with food or images of food—our refrigerators, that candy bowl at work, billboards and food stands on the streets we drive and walk down, cooking shows, food blogs. The quantity that bombards us is unprecedented, and our brains were not designed to resist it. In fact, seeing food makes our brain secrete chemicals that cause cravings, even if our bodies aren't truly hungry.

What the Science Says: What You See Is What You Eat

A Cornell University study compared people who had a clear bowl containing candy on their desk with people who had a white bowl. The candy in the clear bowl was visible; the candy in the white bowl was not. People with a clear candy bowl ate 71 percent more candy than those with a white bowl. As animals whose primary sense is visual, human beings have a physiological response to seeing food or pictures of food. Neurochemically, we anticipate eating it, and our brains start secreting chemicals that cause cravings and can lead to overeating. In addition, people who are obese tend to be more vulnerable to visual cues than normal-weight people.

Food companies know this. In the last several decades, fast food and unhealthy but alluring convenience foods have flourished. The United States leads the world in processed-food consumption. By some estimates, processed foods now make up some 70 percent of Americans' diet, on average. What's more, the quality of American packaged food is exceptionally grim, a landscape of frozen meals, boxed cereals, and sweet and salty snacks that are highly processed, lacking in nutrients, and laden with refined carbohydrates and sugar, unhealthy fats, and chemical additives. (By comparison, many packaged foods in Japan and parts of Europe are less processed, with fewer additives.) The beverage landscape is no better, with Americans consuming sweetened drinks in greater quantities than ever.

Eating convenience food every now and then isn't a problem, but when done regularly, it's extremely harmful to our health. There's a direct link between overconsuming convenience foods and beverages and the epidemics of our day: obesity, insulin resistance, type 2 diabetes, heart disease, and even depression.

While resisting *any* food within reach is difficult, many of today's highly processed foods are addictive by design. Beverage and snack-food flavors like "salted caramel mocha" and "cheddar poppin' pretzel" exist nowhere in nature. These products are developed by taste-and-smell researchers, tweaked for flavor, smell, mouthfeel, and appearance, tested on focus groups, refined by market research, and advertised to the hilt.

Here's what the ads leave out: most food companies are not focused on their customers' weight, health, or emotional well-being; they're focused on selling their products. "No one can eat just one . . ." isn't just a slogan—*it's the goal of food companies everywhere,* and they spend millions to achieve it. That's good for their profits—and bad for our collective health and well-being. Taking advantage of our bodies' innate wiring for carbohydrates, fat, and salt—all necessary for survival when consumed in natural forms and amounts—food companies create products designed to hit what's known as the "bliss point," the combination of flavors and texture that makes a food nearly impossible to stop eating. For them, the less you stop and think, the better. And it's working. One survey found that the amount Americans spend on these highly processed foods nearly doubled from 1982 to 2012, from 11.6 percent to 22.9 percent of our grocery money.

The result of being bombarded by all this packaged food? In terms of sheer availability, eating unhealthy food has never been easier. And healthy eating has never been more elusive.

Profits versus Health

An article published in the journal *Diabetes Care* showed that nine leading brands spent $3.5 billion in a single year to advertise fast food in print and on billboards, TV, and radio. Another $5.8 billion was spent on advertising sweetened drinks, candy, and other food. That's $9.3 billion total—just on advertising. For the same year, the entire budgets for the Centers for Disease Control and Prevention and the Food and Drug Administration were $5.1 billion and $1.3 billion, respectively.

Modifying our immediate environments, to the extent that we can, can help to reduce mindless eating and encourage healthier food choices—you'll learn those strategies here. But to really get a handle on your habits, it's crucial to consider your inner landscape, too.

The Chemistry of Comfort Eating

Food isn't simply physical fuel, nor should it be. We eat to celebrate, we eat for comfort, we eat for pleasure. This has been true throughout history. But in an environment where food abounds and stress levels soar, eating for emotional reasons has become a daily pattern for many people. We use food to fill voids, to obtain instant gratification or stimulation, and to soothe unpleasant feelings such as anxiety, anger, sadness, and stress—whether consciously or unconsciously. For many people, food is a quick fix for emotional pain and a quick filler for emptiness.

We're not just talking about fuzzy feelings; biochemical reactions underpin these cravings. When we feel prolonged stress, our bodies churn out hormones such as cortisol, which cause cravings—for high-sugar

Insights and Inspirations: Daria, age 38

I'm two years into a sales job that requires a lot of travel, and I've gained 17 pounds in that time. That's a lot for anyone, but I'm five-foot-one! There's the obvious fact of having trouble finding anything besides fast food and buffets on the road. But there's also the loneliness factor. At the end of a long day, my husband isn't there to help me wind down. Room service and Netflix are. And on the nights when I'm entertaining clients, we go to high-end restaurants, and there's a certain pressure to spend big and eat big. Steaks, foie gras, expensive wine. Ordering just an appetizer or a salad entrée doesn't feel like an option.

and high-fat foods, in particular. These foods—potato chips, chocolate, cookies, candy, and sweet drinks—trigger a near-immediate calming effect by raising serotonin and dopamine levels. But this eating pattern, over time, sets the stage for weight gain and chronic illness. You'll learn about the chemistry of comfort eating—and how to break the cycle—throughout the book.

A Road Map for Change: Attention + Intention

In working with hundreds of patients on losing weight and changing their eating habits, we've found that two big pieces of the puzzle are often missing from conventional approaches: attention and intention, both infused with the qualities of curiosity and kindness.

Both our culture and our internal selves lead us to automatic, inattentive eating. Attention is one of the keys to stopping that vicious cycle. Paying attention on purpose—tuning in to what's going on in your body, and in your mind, and in the world around you—is at the heart of mindfulness practice, which you'll be learning a lot more about as you progress through the program.

People who have repeatedly tried to lose weight or change eating habits are very familiar with wanting to change but may not be familiar with deep intention. We can spend years, even decades, on the surface layer of change—that basic impulse to "be different, now," with all of our energy tentacles reaching outside ourselves for motivation, for a plan, and for a reward: *I need to eat better in order to look like that blond, willowy beauty over there; I'm going to follow so-and-so's lose-10-pounds-by-bikini-season eating plan; others will find me attractive when I lose the weight.* While external rewards can help people try new things, true, lasting change is different. It emerges from the inside out, not the outside in. This requires reeling in those tentacles and looking within. Lasting change begins with deep intention, alignment between what we deeply value and what we do on a moment-to-moment basis each day of our lives.

In chapter 3, you'll begin a daily mindfulness practice that will help you cultivate both your attention and intention. But today, start with the simple exercises below that introduce these two core concepts. The focus of the first exercise is attention—using your senses and your awareness to notice what is happening around you and within you. This process will prime your brain to create new pathways for behaving differently.

Exercise: Cultivating Attention

As you go about your day, check in with your senses and your mind as described below, as if you were a detective. Hold a curious attitude, looking for clues in your own experiences without criticizing what you observe.

1. Look around. What do you see? Imagine that you have never been in the space you are in right now. How would you describe it to someone who has never been there? Meditators call this "beginner's mind." It involves taking a brand-new perspective.

2. Now close your eyes and listen. What do you hear going on around you? Anything else?

3. Now breathe in deeply. What do you smell?

4. Now, move to the sensations in your body. How does your body feel overall? How do your feet feel? How about your shoulders? How does your stomach feel?

5. And what about your mind? What is it doing right now? Thinking? Planning? Worrying? Making judgments?

Do this three times each day for the next four to five days—morning, afternoon, and night—and pay attention to what you are experiencing. Don't try to change anything; just notice what you see, hear, smell, feel, and think. At the end of each day, write in your journal about your experience. You are beginning to train your mind in how to find important information within yourself.

~

After you've spent a few days practicing *attention*, do the next exercise. In this one, you'll begin to cultivate *intention* by developing a positive image—a "best self." As you progress through the program, you'll be drawn toward it like a magnet.

Exercise: Cultivating Intention

Figuring out what you really want—your deep intention—is a process. If the prospect of deep change is scary to you, that's okay and very common. For now, just notice it and try to get curious about it, keeping in mind that fear can be a form of excitement. To begin, start with this exercise on visualizing your best self, writing your observations down in your journal.

1. Imagine that you are sitting high on a hill, looking out through the distance of time, into the future. You see a shape that looks familiar. As you allow your focus to improve, you slowly realize that this shape is you, five years from now, as your very best self. As the picture becomes clearer, what do you notice? Where are you? What are you doing? How are you feeling? Who else, if anyone, is there with you?

2. When you are done imagining your best self, wave "see you soon" and allow the image to fade. Take a moment now to note your observations:

    What did you notice about your best self?
    What did you notice about the environment around
      your best self?
    How does your best self feel emotionally?
    How does your best self feel physically?
    What has your best self done to get where it is?
    How do you take care of your best self?

Not Perfect, but Present

It's important to note that your best self does *not* mean your "perfect" self. The goal of this program isn't to learn to eat "perfectly." Not only is perfection a myth that's unattainable in real life; perfectionism is counterproductive to change. When your goal is perfection, anything less is a failure. So let's trade in all our ideas about perfection—a perfect diet, a perfect body, a perfect life—for something attainable, real, and useful.

At our clinic, and in this book, we focus not on being perfect, but on being present. What does that mean? When you're present, you're not on autopilot. You begin to understand the cascade of external and internal triggers—everything from food advertising, to being overly hungry, to feeling stressed or lonely—that normally lead to overeating or eating unhealthy food. You're aware of how your body feels, what your thoughts are, and how you're feeling emotionally. Being present means you're able to consciously choose what to eat, when to eat, and how much to eat—and you're aware of why you're eating. Once you establish that inner foundation of presence, you're able to build a sustainable diet that fuels good health, a balanced weight, and happiness.

CHAPTER 2

What's on Your Plate?

"Freedom from obsession is not about something you do; it's about knowing who you are. It's about recognizing what sustains you and what exhausts you."

—Geneen Roth, *Women, Food, and God*

After a decade of "weight creep" in which she gained about 5 pounds a year, Jessica's blood pressure had risen to the point that it was compromising her health. She was determined to lose weight when she made an appointment with one of our nutritionists—she had a legal pad out and was ready to take notes on what and how much to eat. "My doctor says I need to lose 40 pounds," she said. "How long do you think that will take?"

When we did our intake with Jessica, we asked not only about her eating habits, but also about her life. We learned that she had three boys—ages 4 to 12—and that she worked as a reading specialist in the school system. She was a valued employee who was always asked to do more—on committees and projects and fundraisers—and she always said yes, even when it meant skimping on sleep or canceling plans with friends. She was also very involved in her church and her community. "I love my life," she said. But she also said she was "tired all the time" and that all of her commitments got in the way of eating well and exercising.

The fact that Jessica had come to a nutritionist instead of jumping on a diet bandwagon was great. But like a lot of people, she had tunnel vision. When people are focused like a laser beam on the numbers on the scale, we encourage them to step back and widen their gaze, because there's always a bigger picture at work. We've seen in our clinic, again and again, that unhealthy eating habits and excessive weight are never a person's main problem. They're a symptom of some other issue or imbalance.

Our eating habits don't exist in isolation; they exist in the context of our lives. What's on your plate at mealtimes has a lot to do with "what's on your plate"—what's going on in your life. For people like Jessica and so many others, the first step is realizing that those metaphorical plates—their lives—are piled way too high. Taking a step back and assessing the big picture of your life—the whole you—can provide essential perspective about what's going on and what needs to change.

So Much to Do, So Little Time

For many of us, time is in short supply. Life seems to move faster than ever within the same stubborn twenty-four hours, and we're in a constant state of struggling to keep up. We're always multitasking. In a culture that celebrates being "crazy busy" and seems to expect it, we juggle jobs and families, caretaking for children and parents, involvement with community organizations, socializing with friends, and maintaining homes and cars and calendars.

Over the last decade, we've pushed the envelope even further. Staying constantly connected to our jobs and our social circles through our phones and computers has profoundly affected our sense of free time—to say nothing of the social-media explosion. We now feel pressure to stay in touch with not only our families, friends, and coworkers, but also our high-school friends, first loves, far-flung relatives, former colleagues—essentially everyone we've ever known. Whether you find this increasing interconnectedness miraculous or disastrous, or both, it's important to realize how much time—and attention—it requires.

When we look at all the demands on our time and attention, is it any wonder that healthy eating often gets lost in the shuffle? When you're stressed and frazzled, it's hard to pay attention to what's going on in your body—we'll delve into that in chapter 5. But on a more basic level, unless you're blessed with a personal chef, eating well takes time: planning time, shopping time, cooking time, and time to eat slowly and consciously. When you're trying to change your habits, you also need time to get to know yourself.

Making space for eating better, then, requires reckoning with the fact that you are a human being with a finite amount of time and energy. You might have to remind yourself of this reality *repeatedly*, since so many aspects of our lives push against it. The next step is seeing how you currently allocate those precious resources—your time and energy—and how different aspects of your life affect your eating habits.

Connecting the Dots

Determining what in your life needs changing and how to make those changes is not always obvious. And even when it becomes clear, the prospect of making changes can be overwhelming. At Duke IM we've developed an illustrative tool that's helped thousands of people gain clarity about the changes they wish to make. Called the Wheel of Health (see page 28 for an illustration), it's based on the idea that health—including eating and exercise habits—does not exist in isolation. Health is not something that exists only in our bodies, separate from our lives. Rather, health is *deeply intertwined* with every aspect of our lives.

If your work life is busy and stressful, for instance, you may opt for takeout more and postpone your exercise plans. If you don't have a lot of intimacy in your life, you might use food as a substitute for close relationships. If you've been overweight for a long time, you might experience back pain or joint pain, which makes you reluctant to exercise. You might have negative feelings about your body, which affect your relationships, or you might feel stigmatized at work—53 percent of overweight people say they do.

Normally, the different aspects of our lives are swirling so fast we aren't aware of which parts are functioning well and which aren't, let alone how they affect one another. Weight gain and unhealthy habits such as chronic overeating occur for many reasons, but most have to do with having too many commitments elsewhere in life that trump taking care of your body. The Wheel of Health—divided into seven domains, with mindful awareness at the center (described on page 34)—helps you step back and assess those commitments, to pause and really look at how you spend your time and energy. Very often, some areas of the wheel are overflowing while others are empty; such imbalances drain our energy.

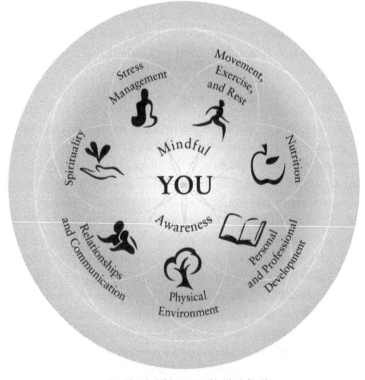

Time and again, patients in our clinic have "a-ha" moments as they assess different areas of their lives and see how issues or imbalances may be affecting their eating habits. Many people realize that they're spending so much time working, there's little left for healthy eating and exercise (to say nothing of the biochemical effects of chronic stress, which often accompanies overwork). Relationship issues, ranging from marriage problems to loneliness to difficulty communicating one's feelings, are another common thread.

For some people, taking stock of their personal Wheel of Health is not as much of an "a-ha" moment as a reckoning. They might know full well what areas of their life are affecting their eating habits but feel unable to change them. Melissa, a young woman who visited our clinic, had gradually gained about 15 pounds over the last three years. Her diet was fairly healthy, but she had developed a habit of eating a large bowl of ice cream after dinner every night before bed. When asked if she knew how that habit started, she nodded and said, "Every Saturday night when I was a kid, my dad and I would watch a movie and eat ice cream. Butter pecan." Her dad had died three years ago unexpectedly, and eating ice cream comforted her and helped her feel connected to him. She didn't

Insights and Inspirations: Lisa, age 39

I got a promotion four years ago and started traveling for work a lot. It meant a lot more money, which was exciting, and for a while I felt like I was on the top of my game. But my health started to suffer. I had to start taking sleeping pills because my body felt so wacked out from changing time zones, and I was too tired to even try to exercise or eat well. My friends, who had always been a source of strength for me, started to feel like abstractions because I was never home. Then my dad got sick. That's when it hit me that I had to stop traveling, which was a scary idea. Ultimately I switched to a different company and took a pay cut. That was a tough decision, but my health and my life have been getting better ever since.

want to lose that connection. It made a lot of sense. We worked with her on how to cherish the memories of her dad in a way that supported her health goals instead of undermining them. As it turned out, he had been an avid hiker, and Melissa liked the idea of incorporating a hike into her weekend routine. She also decided to cut back on her ice-cream habit but not eliminate it—having a small bowl once a week.

Exploring your Wheel of Health forces you to slow down and get a bird's-eye view of your life.

In the following exercise, you will use the Wheel of Health to guide you in assessing the big picture of your life. Remember that *you know your life better than anyone else*. Your own insight will go a long way toward helping you identify areas that are out of balance, and which of those areas you will be most successful at changing. And as you read the book, you'll learn more about each area, how it can contribute to your eating habits, and how to make improvements.

Exercise: Your Wheel of Health

1. Draw and label your own Wheel of Health in your journal.

2. Read through the seven areas of health described below, as well as the description of the Wheel of Health's center—mindful awareness. The questions in each section will help you assess how well you're doing within each area; write the answers in your journal. Using these answers as a guide, you'll consider how satisfied you are with how well you're taking care of yourself, and give yourself a rating of 1 to 10 in each area.

Stress management. Chronic stress takes an enormous toll on our health and happiness and contributes to unhealthy eating. While we won't ever eliminate stress, managing it is essential for good physical and mental

Your Wheel of Health

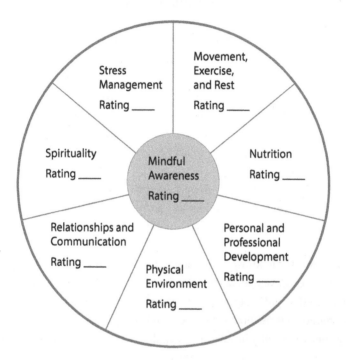

health. *How much stress are you experiencing right now? Over the last three months, six months, year? How well do you think you are managing/coping with the stress in your life? Do you feel as if your body is always revved up, waiting for the next problem to develop? Do you think you have enough coping strategies, or would you benefit from learning additional strategies? Are you using the strategies you have effectively? Do you have a regular activity that you practice that makes you feel relaxed?*

How satisfied are you with how well you're taking care of yourself in this area? Give yourself a rating of 1 to 10, with 1 being "not satisfied" and 10 being "extremely satisfied." Add the rating to your wheel.

Movement, exercise, and rest. Our bodies were designed to move, and we know that exercise is required for optimal health. It is also required to maintain optimal metabolism and to manage weight for the long run. However, it's easy to become sedentary with all of the conveniences of modern life. We may not carve out and protect time for exercise or movement, and we may not even be checking in with our bodies to notice how they want and need to move. We also need rest—deep rest during sleep, and mental rest even when awake. *Do you lead an active life? How much do you move your body? Do you consciously include physical activities in your daily life? Do you engage in planned aerobic exercise regularly? Do you include strength training in your exercise? Do you allow yourself downtime to rest? Do you give yourself plenty of time to unwind before bed? How refreshing is your sleep?*

How satisfied are you with how well you're taking care of yourself in this area? Give yourself a rating of 1 to 10, with 1 being "not satisfied" and 10 being "extremely satisfied." Add the rating to your wheel.

Nutrition. The foods we eat—and beverages we drink—profoundly affect our health and well-being. There's a direct connection between the quality of the food we put in our bodies and our energy levels, our immune health, our moods, our risk of chronic illness, and, of course, our weight. Nourishing our bodies with a healthy diet (including vegetables, healthy fats, whole grains, fruit, and lean proteins) provides a foundation for good health. *Do you know what to eat to keep your body as healthy as possible? To maintain good energy? Do you eat those healthy foods? And in appropriate amounts? Are there things that you're doing well and want to maintain regarding your eating? Are there things that you know you would benefit from changing?*

How satisfied are you with how well you're taking care of yourself in this area? Give yourself a rating of 1 to 10, with 1 being "not satisfied" and 10 being "extremely satisfied." Add the rating to your wheel.

Personal and professional development. Our work lives have an impact on our health in myriad ways, including the ways in which they tax us and the ways in which they fulfill us. Work-life balance is important, and lacking for some people. Additionally, continued learning keeps people engaged and alive. Some people find this at work, some through education, and some through pursuing other interests. What's important is that you find it somewhere. It's also important to live your life according to your values and priorities. Balance in this area of health may be about the number of work hours you put in or the amount of effort you put forth, or it may be more about how fulfilling your work is, the amount of praise or respect you receive at work, the degree of autonomy you have in doing your work, or the significance of the impact you create. *Do you feel satisfied or fulfilled in your life—at home and at work? Do you have an acceptable work–life balance? Are there areas to explore that might give you a deeper sense of motivation and joy in your life? Are there small changes that you could make to increase your sense of purpose, growth, and meaningfulness in your life? Do you make time for enjoyable activities—the things you love to do, or have dreams of doing?*

How satisfied are you with how well you're taking care of yourself in this area? Give yourself a rating of 1 to 10, with 1 being "not satisfied" and 10 being "extremely satisfied." Add the rating to your wheel.

Physical environment. Your surroundings can influence your health in many ways, including affecting your eating habits. If your pantry and fridge are filled with unhealthy snacks and sweets, for example, you're much more likely to eat those foods—whereas if you have fresh produce and other healthy foods on hand, you're more likely to reach for those. It is important to give some thought to how your environment can support your health. It's also important to consider how your space makes you feel. For some people, excessive noise or clutter can be stressful, which can in turn affect eating and exercise habits. *Is your home set up to facilitate healthy eating? How about your workplace? Do your home and work space make you feel relaxed or stressed? Is there sufficient natural light? Do you have concerns about noise or clutter?*

How satisfied are you with how well you're taking care of yourself in this area? Give yourself a rating of 1 to 10, with 1 being "not satisfied" and 10 being "extremely satisfied." Add the rating to your wheel.

Relationships and communication. Positive connections with others enhance not only your quality of life, but also your health. Not being able to communicate your needs or feeling uncomfortable saying "no" to others can lead to frustration, resentment, or unnecessary self-sacrifice. This is true in all relationships—romantic relationships as well as those with friends, family, and coworkers. *How would you describe your relationships with others and your communication with them? Are your needs met? Are you helping others meet theirs? Do you have a few key people with whom you can share the more intimate details of your life, or just blow off some steam and have a few laughs with? Are you able to ask for support and let the people in your life know what you wish them to do or not do in support of you? Are there certain relationships that drain you and others that nourish you?*

How satisfied are you with how well you're taking care of yourself in this area? Give yourself a rating of 1 to 10, with 1 being "not satisfied" and 10 being "extremely satisfied." Add the rating to your wheel.

Spirituality. Spiritual connections offer positive effects on health and well-being, and give people a sense of meaning, peace, and inspiration. Some people are drawn to formal religious practice and prayer. Others find a sense of peace and spiritual connection by spending time in nature. *Do you have a spiritual practice, or a place you go that makes you feel renewed and helps you connect to something larger than yourself? Are there meaningful rituals in your life?*

How satisfied are you with how well you're taking care of yourself in this area? Give yourself a rating of 1 to 10, with 1 being "not satisfied" and 10 being "extremely satisfied." Add the rating to your wheel.

Mindful awareness. Mindful awareness sits at the center of the Wheel of Health and offers us the opportunity to be more in touch with our bodies, our minds, and the spiritual aspects of self—our internal worlds that we often ignore. Mindful awareness is central to the hard and rewarding work of getting to know yourself on a deeper level. You'll use your own deep wisdom to help you change eating habits and other behavior patterns. Mindful awareness implies an ability to be fully present in the moment, paying attention to what you are doing while you are doing it. It means fully experiencing and attending to what is happening—not only outside of you but, more important, *within* you. Mindfulness also helps you to be conscious of what is truly important to you. *How aware are you of how your body feels at each moment? Of emotions you have at each moment? Of thoughts that run through your mind? Of needs that drive your behavior? Of how you are interacting with the outside world? How much do you pay attention to what's going on inside of you from moment to moment?*

How satisfied are you with how well you're taking care of yourself in this area? Give yourself a rating of 1 to 10; add it to your wheel. This area may be new to you. If you are not sure how to rate it, don't worry; you will be able to better assess it once you better understand and have begun to practice mindfulness as you progress through this book.

∼

Now it's time to look at your Wheel of Health as a whole and consider where to start making changes. Review your responses. Can you draw connections between imbalances in your life and your eating habits? Are other commitments in your life crowding out your time to prepare healthy food, for instance? Or do you have a sense that you are eating to compensate for a lack of fulfillment in other areas? Look at the areas with the lowest satisfaction ratings, and among those, pick an area that's particularly meaningful to you. Rather than starting with a major change, think about a small change you can make. Suppose you gave yourself a "4" in stress management and you have a sense that your typically harried lifestyle is what keeps you from preparing healthy food each night. Or say you gave yourself a "3" in movement, exercise, and rest because you don't exercise regularly—but you want to. Rather than signing up for a 10K, plan to start walking with a friend three times a week. (You'll learn more about setting goals for sustainable change in the next chapter.)

Insights and Inspirations: Sandy, age 52

I've been trying to lose weight since I was 12 years old. When I looked at the relationship area of my life, it was empty, and had been since my divorce ten years ago. I wish I could say it's a coincidence that I've gained a lot of weight during that time, but it's not. I know it's not. Getting back out there, trying to find a new intimate relationship, is scary. But I have a feeling that's part of what I really need.

The good thing about eating and life being so intertwined is that it leaves us with many options of where to start "untangling" ourselves and restructure our lives to be our best selves. Achieving balance is a dance—a dynamic process, not a static one. When you come to terms with the fact that eating is one component in the wheel of your whole life, with each component creating ripple effects back and forth, you realize that changing your eating habits is going to entail making changes in your life. In other words, you're going to have to shake things up. This might excite you, or frighten you, or both. We tend to be comfortable with the status quo, even when it's not supporting our health. As one of our clients put it, "It might be a crazy life, but it's *my* crazy life!" That feeling is normal, and the important thing is to see it for what it is—our desire to stay in our comfort zone. When our comfort zone is at odds with our health—and it often is—we have some decisions to make. It's a process, but that's what *The Mindful Diet* is about—giving you the tools to work through that process.

The Starting Block: Self-Care

The Wheel of Health can help you discern the best places to focus first in achieving a healthier balance between the different areas of your life. Self-care is critical to achieving that balance. Many of us, women especially, spend a lot of time taking care of people and things—families, work, households, finances. Taking care of ourselves often feels like indulgence. Or maybe it's something you'd do if you had time for it, but you never do.

If taking good care of yourself feels selfish, consider the possibility that self-care is the fuel that makes all other care and all other life activities possible. It makes life sustainable. *Self-care is not self-indulgence; it's self-preservation.* If that message strikes a chord with you, write it down where you can see it—on a chalkboard at home, on your fridge, or on a sticky note taped to your computer. Even if you've lost touch with it, consider that there's a piece of you that knows, deep down, what is healthy for you, that knows your best self, the one that you envisioned in chapter 1. And it doesn't just *know* what's healthy, it *wants* what's healthy: a long walk instead of a hot-fudge sundae, a reasonable work schedule instead of a sixty-hour week, more time laughing with friends instead of the fleeting pleasure offered by French fries at the drive-through.

Insights and Inspirations: Lauren, age 35

My pattern for years was to get an egg sandwich and two hash browns on the way to work and eat in the car. I looked forward to it and figured I was killing two birds with one stone. When I started paying attention, I noticed that I always had a greasy lump in my stomach all morning—and it dawned on me that a third of my meals were coming from fast food! My biggest realization, though, was that part of taking care of myself was carving out time to prepare healthy food. I'd always thought of "me time" as a pedicure, or going out for drinks with friends—something that felt indulgent. But getting up twenty minutes earlier to make and eat breakfast turned out to be this amazing thing. I got some quiet time in the house before the kids got up, my commute was less frantic, and I felt so much better. The greasy lump disappeared, and I had more energy.

Quiz: How's your self-care?

I do the following . . .	rarely	some- times	often
Sit down to eat meals	❑	❑	❑
Get seven to nine hours of sleep most nights and wake feeling rested	❑	❑	❑
Have a relaxing bedtime routine	❑	❑	❑
Take breaks during my workday to recharge	❑	❑	❑
Seek out emotional support when I need it	❑	❑	❑
Make time to enjoy myself	❑	❑	❑
Say no to requests that aren't right for me	❑	❑	❑
Schedule time to "play" with friends	❑	❑	❑
Make time to prepare healthy meals	❑	❑	❑
Schedule dates with my spouse or partner	❑	❑	❑
Let my body move as it was meant to, doing physical activity each day	❑	❑	❑
Do planned aerobic exercise at least four times a week	❑	❑	❑
Regularly invest time in something that helps me grow and develop some aspect of myself	❑	❑	❑
Take care of the space around me (home, kitchen, work), in order to support my goals	❑	❑	❑

Circle anything that you scored as "rarely." When it comes to making changes, these will be important areas to consider—and whether or not they're directly related to eating, they'll help to *support* healthy eating and overall health.

~

You don't have to know what good self-care looks like right now, or how the balance of your life might need to change, or exactly what and how much you should be eating. But know this: *good self-care is essential for changing what, why, and how you eat.* And more important, it's essential for changing how satisfied, balanced, and fulfilled you feel in your life.

Building Your Foundation: Your Values

Assessing what's on your plate—in both the literal and figurative senses—is one thing; making changes is another. Your innermost values can serve as an important guide. Getting in touch with your values supports what psychologists call **intrinsic motivation,** motivation that comes from within. Research shows that new eating and exercise habits are much more likely to stick when they spring from within us rather than from external sources. Thinking about your core values can be a useful way to create sustainable health goals, which you'll learn more about at the end of chapter 3. Keeping your values in mind can also help you make moment-to-moment decisions about eating, exercise, life balance, and self-care.

Exercise: Knowing Your Core Values

1. Make a list in your journal with three columns: Very Important to Me, Important to Me, and Not at All Important to Me. (Depending on the size of your journal, you may need one to several pages.) Review the following list of personal values and assign each of them to one of the columns.

Personal Values

Acceptance (to be accepted as I am)
Accuracy (to be accurate in my opinions and beliefs)
Achievement (to have important accomplishments)
Adventure (to have new and exciting experiences)
Attractiveness (to be physically attractive)
Authority (to be in charge of and responsible for others)
Autonomy (to be self-determined and independent)
Beauty (to appreciate beauty around me)
Caring (to take care of others)
Comfort (to have a pleasant and comfortable life)
Commitment (to make enduring, meaningful commitments)
Compassion (to feel and act on concern for others)

Complexity (to have a life full of variety and change)
Contribution (to make a lasting contribution to the world)
Courtesy (to be considerate and polite toward others)
Creativity (to have new and original ideas)
Dependability (to be reliable and trustworthy)
Duty (to carry out my duties and obligations)
Ecology (to live in harmony with the environment)
Faithfulness (to be loyal and true in relationships)
Fame (to be known and recognized)
Family (to have a happy, loving family)
Flexibility (to adjust to new circumstances easily)
Forgiveness (to be forgiving of others)
Friendship (to have close, supportive friends)
Fun (to play and have fun)
Generosity (to give what I have to others)
Genuineness (to act in a manner that is true to who I am)
Growth (to keep changing and growing)
Health and well-being (to be physically and mentally well
    and healthy)
Helpfulness (to be helpful to others)
Honesty (to be honest and truthful)
Hope (to maintain a positive and optimistic outlook)
Humility (to be modest and unassuming)
Humor (to see the humorous side of myself and the world)
Independence (to be free from dependence on others)
Industry (to work hard and well at my life tasks)
Inner Peace (to experience personal peace)
Intimacy (to share my innermost experiences with others)
Justice (to promote fair and equal treatment for all)
Knowledge (to learn and contribute)
Leisure (to take time to relax and enjoy)
Logic (to live rationally and sensibly)
Loved (to be loved by those close to me)
Loving (to give love to others)
Mastery (to be competent in everyday or specialized activities)
Moderation (to avoid excesses and find a middle ground)

Monogamy (to have one close, loving relationship)
Order (to have a life that is well-ordered and organized)
Pleasure (to feel good)
Popularity (to be well-liked by many people)
Power (to have control over others)
Purpose (to have meaning and direction in my life)
Realism (to see and act realistically and practically)
Responsibility (to make and carry out responsible decisions)
Risk (to take risks and chances)
Romance (to have intense, exciting love in my life)
Safety (to be safe and secure)
Self-Acceptance (to accept myself as I am)
Self-Control (to be disciplined in my own actions)
Self-Knowledge (to have a deep and honest understanding
    of myself)
Service (to be of service to others)
Simplicity (to live life simply, with minimal needs)
Spirituality (to grow and mature spiritually)
Stability (to have a life that stays fairly consistent)
Strength (to be physically fit and strong)
Tolerance (to accept and respect those who differ from me)
Tradition (to follow respected patterns of the past)
Virtue (to live a morally sound life)
Wealth (to have plenty of money)
World Peace (to work to promote peace in the world)
Other Value(s)

2. After you've grouped all of these values by importance,
   look only at those in the "Very Important" column. On a
   separate page, or in the space below, write the five or six
   values from this column that are of *utmost* importance to
   you. Feel free to choose different words if they fit better
   for you. These are your core values. If there's a core value
   not listed here, feel free to add it. And keep in mind that it
   takes some people a while to narrow down their values to
   the most important few. So if it feels impossible to narrow
   it down, come back to this exercise later.

3. Now reflect on your health. How does your health relate to what you most value? Were health and well-being in your top five values? Are they qualities you need in order to manifest or live your top five? For instance, if adventure is one of your core values, staying in good physical condition (health) is important.

Sustainable Change Takes "The Whole You"

As you've seen in this chapter, healthful eating doesn't just happen; it takes time, energy, and attention—and connecting to your deeper self. So improving your eating habits—and improving your life—requires making changes. For Jessica, the overcommitted mother of three boys, assessing her Wheel of Health and doing the values exercise helped her to recognize that service and family were two of her core values. She realized that she was spreading herself so thin that she didn't feel fully present in any area of her life; she was always rushing and thinking about the next commitment. And while health was *not* one of her core values, she needed it to keep up with her three boys; the extra weight she gained was making it hard to do bike rides and other activities with them.

As you progress through the program, notice how making changes to what's on your plate in the metaphorical sense influences what ends up on your literal plate. Repeat the Wheel of Health exercise every three to six months to get a bird's-eye view of your life. Think of your values as your home base—the place you return to. As you'll see, keeping your values in mind—at the forefront instead of in the background—will help you make moment-to-moment decisions about eating, exercise, and self-care. It will also help you develop realistic goals that support your health. But first, you'll learn how to dismantle the *unrealistic* goals that our diet-obsessed culture imposes on all of us—and learn how to recognize the influence of the diet industry on the ways we think about food, our bodies, and change itself.

CHAPTER 3

Getting Off the Roller Coaster

"[T]o promise not to do a thing is the surest way in the world to make a body want to go and do that very thing."

—Mark Twain, *The Adventures of Tom Sawyer*

With nearly 70 percent of Americans now overweight or obese, products and programs that claim to help people lose weight have become ever more popular. Every year, more than 100 million Americans go on a diet—spending tens of billions on weight-loss plans and books, diet drugs and supplements, and diet-labeled meals and drinks.

Diet programs keep quiet about the fact that they thrive on failure. Many people who diet lose weight initially, but studies show that the vast majority—more than 80 percent—gain it back within five years, and many seesaw for decades. And for reasons that scientists are just beginning to understand, many people who lose weight on a diet gain it all back and then some, ending up heavier and less healthy than overweight people who never dieted in the first place.

The psychology of dieting may be the most damaging of all, and it affects all of us—dieters and nondieters alike. Having been part of our societal landscape for decades, diet-related thought patterns undermine the eating habits of all of us. What's more, the diet mentality and the diet industry have hijacked the whole notion of change. The just-do-it, power-through-it, all-or-nothing approach to changing our habits, with motivation coming from outside oneself, ignores the key to authentic, lasting change: YOU. **To forge a healthy relationship with food and your body, you need to recognize the diet mentality for what it is—a misleading promise that sets you up to fail—and begin the process of changing from within.**

A Losing Formula

Typical weight-loss diets work—in the short term—by restricting calories. Naturally, this leaves you wanting more food. And while you may be able to tolerate hunger for a finite period of time, few people can do so long-term. In fact, restricting calories often leads to overeating, or even bingeing. This isn't a failure of willpower; it's our survival instincts. Human bodies evolved to cope with famine, and when we restrict food, our brain sends out urgent signals to eat in the form of ghrelin, a hormone that stimulates appetite. Evidence shows that is exactly what happens with restrictive diets, so it's no wonder they backfire.

Even diets that provide your body with a sufficient number of calories may leave you wanting more. Extreme low-fat diets, for instance, tend to be unsatisfying for most people for the simple reason that dietary fat (along with protein) helps your body feel full, because it takes your body longer to digest fat than to digest carbohydrates. What happens when we don't feel satisfied? Very often we keep eating. And there goes the diet.

The Diet Seduction (and Betrayal)

Many people try to lose weight for decades and, not surprisingly, feel frustrated at their lack of success and desperate for something, *anything*, that works. When you're struggling with weight loss, it's easy to fall prey to slogans and promises that may not be honest but are music to your ears: *Stop your eating struggles now! Eat whatever you want and never feel hungry! We have a magic formula for weight loss!*

Diet companies' marketing tactics often play into body insecurities, with promises that you'll get your "best body," shed 20 pounds by bikini season, or lose your baby belly, and plentiful visuals of the alleged end results. The message that there's a thin, toned, youthful body inside you waiting to break free—that this is, in fact, the *real* you—is a hallmark of popular diets. Often they claim to target specific body parts—for women, most often it's the belly, thighs, or butt, places where our bodies naturally store extra fat and about which many of us harbor negative feelings. (We'll delve more deeply into how our relationship with our bodies affects our eating habits—and vice versa—in chapter 8.)

Not all popular diets are blatantly irresponsible. But even the "better" ones, with nutritionally sound plans, tend to fail. It's not just the particulars of a given diet that are problematic—it's the very psychology of dieting.

Most structured diet plans have a simple and seductive message: eat these foods, in these amounts, and you'll lose weight. The underlying assumption is that the solution to out-of-control eating is to clamp down on it, with *hyper*-controlled eating. There's an obvious appeal to this approach. When you're struggling to eat healthy foods in healthy amounts, surrendering to an outside authority that tells you exactly what to do can feel like a huge relief. And dieting can be a tangible focus and strategy amid life issues that are too overwhelming or complicated to tackle (and sometimes even to acknowledge). People often look to weight loss as their holy grail. *If I lose weight, the rest of my life will sort itself out,* the thinking goes. In fact, it's often the other way around, as you learned in exploring your Wheel of Health.

Despite its appeal, relying on an outside authority—**external motivation**—sets you up to fail. As we mentioned in the last chapter, research shows that **internal motivation** is required for long-term, sustainable behavior change. When you follow a prescriptive plan, you don't address *why* you're overeating and eating junk in the first place. Without that crucial insight, it's natural, even inevitable, to revert to old habits as soon as you stop following the rules. Whatever diet you're following may temporarily override your usual patterns, but those patterns are alive and well at the end of the diet—and they often reemerge with a vengeance. And given the autopilot nature of eating—the fact that there are myriad triggers for taking that first bite or not stopping when you should—it's no wonder why.

Insights and Inspirations: Judy, age 44

I was stuck on the diet treadmill for years, always starting with gusto and ending in defeat. Then somehow I'd forget how awful I felt at the end and try again, like I had amnesia. The diet let me keep this fantasy going of the person I just knew I'd be when I lost the weight. Not just thin, but more "together," better dressed, and happier—even wealthier! I used to imagine myself wearing one of those strapless dresses that really thin women look great in, the kind that shows off your collarbones. It took up so much of my energy, the whole process—it became this vortex that propelled me—but I never got anywhere. In fact, I felt worse, physically and emotionally. It took me a long time to realize why.

The Diet Mentality (It's Not Just for Dieters)

Diet-related thought patterns have become the cultural norm, and they are especially insidious because they undermine healthy change instead of promoting it. From a psychological point of view, many ideas people hold about food, dieting, weight loss, and our bodies are **cognitive distortions**—unconscious thinking patterns that are not based in reality.

Black-and-white thinking (also called **all-or-nothing thinking**) is a prime cognitive distortion that has become part of our cultural zeitgeist—for example: *there are good foods and bad foods, certain foods are off-limits, you're either a healthy eater or an unhealthy eater, you're* *either "on the wagon" or off it, you should never eat past 8 P.M.* There certainly are healthier choices and less healthy choices, and our program guides you toward the healthier ones. But *why* you're eating matters, even if you're eating healthy food. When you base your plans on rigid rules, it's virtually impossible not to break them at some point. **Catastrophizing,** a cognitive distortion that often accompanies all-or-nothing thinking, happens when you predict that disastrous outcomes will follow from your action or inaction, such as, *I did not exercise this morning . . . therefore, I will never get in shape and I'll be overweight forever.* Perhaps the most pervasive fallacy is the **willpower myth,** the idea that succumbing to unhealthy cravings (or falling off the diet wagon) is a failure of will and a sign of personal weakness. Cultivating willpower *is* important in terms of learning to delay gratification, but it's unrealistic to think it's the only thing needed in our over-the-top food environment.

Katy, age 41, a client who says she's always been a "sugar fiend," consumes a cheese Danish on the way to work most days, candy in the afternoons, and ice cream or cookies at night. In order to gain energy and lose a few pounds, she decides to go cold turkey on anything with refined sugar. She doesn't have a backup plan and does not stop to consider why she's eating so much sugar in the first place. She finds herself thinking about sweets nonstop and criticizing herself for it. But the more she reprimands herself, the more she obsesses. After struggling and fending off sweets for two weeks, she finds herself in a vulnerable situation: overtired and stressed, at an office party where there are platters piled high with cookies, her main weakness. She wants one. She *needs* one. One turns into two, and then three, and then five. Driving home, she harshly berates herself for eating the cookies and feels despairing. She thinks that she's lost all control, not unlike an alcoholic or a smoker who has fallen off the wagon. And there goes her attempt to change her habits. "I'm hopeless. I will never be able to give up sugar," she thinks. She throws in the towel and starts the next morning with a Danish.

We hear stories like Katy's every day. The result of all these punitive, untrue, and unhelpful thought patterns? We set up eating as a battle to be won, but the rules of engagement make "losing" inevitable.

All-or-Nothing Food Groups

On a cultural level, black-and-white thinking about food has demonized entire macronutrients (in particular, carbohydrates and fat), to the detriment of millions of people's health. The low-fat movement that started in the 1970s, based on the misguided hyping of a report linking dietary fat to heart disease, is a prime example. People started avoiding all fat as if it were arsenic but increasing carbohydrates (mostly refined), and the low-fat processed-food industry took off. We'll talk more about the fat fallacy in chapter 10, but to make a long story short, *good* fat is essential for your health—and processed foods that are low in fat but high in refined carbohydrates, calories, and man-made additives are harmful to health. Despite nutritionists' efforts to promote the truth about fat in recent years, emphasizing the difference between healthy and less healthy fats, the black-and-white idea that "fat is bad" has stuck like glue.

The more-recent demonization of carbohydrates, another class of macronutrients that includes both healthy and unhealthy varieties, has also been damaging. As with fat, the truth is not black-and-white. Refined, processed carbohydrates and sugar are indeed unhealthy, but plant sources of carbohydrates such as vegetables, fruit, beans and legumes, and whole grains are important for good health, disease prevention, and physical and mental energy.

The Enemy Within

When you set yourself up with rigid, black-and-white rules to completely abstain from certain foods, there's no room for error. You're either on the diet or you're off it. Once you've had the cookie, you're off the wagon—and that means anything goes. What's the difference between two cookies and twelve? You'll start the sugar ban again next week—or maybe next month.

Here's the worst part: the guilt, shame, and self-criticism that ensue from "breaking the rules" can make you avoid healthy-eating efforts entirely. This might seem like self-sabotage, but it's actually quite rational: If you know that you're going to get punished for failing, why try? Who wants to get punished? In our program, we refer to the self-critical part of ourselves as the **Inner Critic.** It's a harsh inner voice that focuses on only one aspect of ourselves—a weakness for sugar, for example—with a spirit of meanness, without looking at the bigger picture of who we are. The condemnation that the Inner Critic dishes out leads us to feel *worse* and have *less* energy to change. When our learned experience of trying to change our behavior is so painful, we avoid trying. Health psychologists refer to the failure-shame-avoidance spiral that results from breaking rigid rules as the "abstinence violation effect."

Exercise: Diet-related Thought Patterns

One of the tools of mindfulness is noticing. Simply being aware of the traps and tricks of the diet mentality has powerful effects. We'll start developing a daily practice for cultivating awareness in the next chapter, but starting now, make an effort to notice when you're in the grip of the willpower myth, black-and-white thinking, catastrophizing, or deprivation and obsession. Notice when you hear the voice of the Inner Critic. On your calendar or journal, jot down what you notice your mind saying, without making any judgments.

Keep in mind, too, the dance between **deprivation and obsession.** Forbidding yourself to eat a particular food that you really enjoy—chocolate, for example—tends to make you not only crave the food but *obsess* about the food. It's as if someone tells you not to think about the color blue and the word "umbrella." Suddenly, there are blue umbrellas everywhere you look.

The antidote to deprivation is not constant indulgence, but setting limits that still give you freedom of choice.

Health Happens "In the Middle"

It's rare that our days—at work, at home, and everywhere in between—go exactly as planned. Our kids get sick; *we* get sick; we get stuck in traffic; we get bad news about a friend's health; our boss adds an extra project to our overflowing plate. "Life happens," we say in our clinic, meaning that we all face curveballs—large and small—on a regular basis. The healthiest people, psychologically, are flexible—they're able to adapt their behavior to changing circumstances and think in shades of gray, rather than in black and white.

The diet mentality isn't just counterproductive to weight loss and overall health; it runs counter to emotional health, too. Psychologists use the term **cognitive rigidity** to describe thought patterns that are so ingrained that people have trouble thinking flexibly. Human beings are not robots. It's *normal* to have a hard time following a rigid plan—whether it's a diet, a "detox," or a cold-turkey attempt to give up sugar. In order to maintain healthy eating habits in an ever-changing world, flexibility is essential.

For a lot of people who've been struggling with their eating habits, the whole notion of flexibility is scary, bringing to mind an "anything goes" mind-set that will do *anything but* curb their unhealthy habits. And that concern is valid. We are not saying "anything goes." Having ample flexibility but no goals or guidelines can leave us adrift in our attempts to make changes—we don't even know where to start. How, then, do you make changes without getting locked into a rigid plan?

Behavior-change success is most sustainable when people become skillful "in the middle" rather than at the extremes. For changing your eating habits and maintaining those changes, it's important to have goals and guidelines, but also enough flexibility to allow you to adapt to changing circumstances—including getting off track. This runs counter to the diet mentality *and* counter to "anything goes"—and it's sustainable.

What are the differences between rules and guidelines? It's more than semantics. See the chart below for a cheat sheet on the distinctions, and notice too the difference between guidelines and "anything goes."

"Anything Goes"	Guidelines	Rules
Complete lack of structure	Flexible, adaptable structure	Absolute, rigid structure
Wide-open, permissive perspective	Allow for shades of gray—middle ground	Black-and-white perspective
Avoidance of commands and suggestions	Positive and negative suggestions	Often negative ("Don't" commands)
No goals or expectations	Realistic goals and expectations	Unrealistic goals and expectations
Health problems related to unhealthy eating	Sustainable behavior and health	Unsustainable behavior and increased risk of unhealthy eating
Eat as much dessert as you want, whenever you want.	*When you really want dessert, have three bites and savor each one.*	*Never eat dessert.*

Exercise: Flip the Script

Think about where you are on the continuum between having no structure and having rigid structure when it comes to eating. Do you have any rules for yourself? If so, write them down, and spend some time thinking about each one. Where did the rule come from? Does it work for you? How do you feel when you break it? Does it support your health? Finally, think about whether there's a guideline that might take the place of the rule.

If you're more of an "anything goes" person, ask yourself how that came to be. Does it work for you and support your health? How does it make you feel? Are there immediate consequences to "anything goes"? How about long-term consequences? Think of a guideline you'd like to try in order to bring more structure to your eating habits.

Try out your new guideline for a week, see how it works for you, and reflect on it in your journal.

Sample Exercises

Where I am on the continuum: *Rigid*

Example: *I never eat chocolate.*

Rationale: *I am a chocoholic, and if I allow myself any I'll lose control.*

How this plays out: *I stay chocolate-free for days, sometimes weeks, and then binge on candy bars when I'm having a bad day.*

What I tell myself: *I have no willpower. I'm a loser.*

Does being rigid support my health? *No.*

New guideline: *I allow myself a small piece of dark chocolate in the afternoon if I want one.*

How it worked: *I ate too much chocolate the first few days, was excited and didn't quite stick to the guideline. But now it doesn't feel like such a big deal. I even skipped chocolate yesterday.*

Where I am on the continuum: *Anything goes*

Example: *I let myself eat French fries whenever I crave them (which is often).*

Rationale: *Certain foods make me happy, and I'm not going to deny myself that happiness.*

How this plays out: *I end up at the drive-through on the way home from work three or four days a week. It usually gives me a stomachache.*

What I tell myself: *I deserve a little indulgence after a stressful day.*

Does "anything goes" support my health? *No.*

New guideline: *I allow myself a small order of fries every now and then, after checking in with myself about why I want them.*

How it worked: *I feel proud of myself, like I have more restraint, and I know I can still have a treat when I plan for it.*

Insights and Inspirations: Elizabeth, age 48

In my house growing up, fattening foods were the ultimate no-no. No butter, no cheese. Even avocados and olive oil were suspect. My mom kept PAM cooking spray in business. I'd binge on pepperoni pizza and ice cream when my parents weren't around; I couldn't get enough. In hindsight, I wonder if my body needed the fat! One time I went to a friend's house for dinner—she was Italian. Her mom served fresh cheese, vegetables, bread dipped in olive oil, and this amazing fish with fresh herbs. Gelato for dessert. I asked my friend if they ate that way all the time, and she said yes—except for the dessert, which was for special occasions. I might as well have been doing drugs—that's how I felt on my way home. I told my mom we had baked chicken and steamed green beans so she'd let me go back.

Get Moving Mindfully

Like healthy food, physical activity (and the lack of it) plays an enormous role in our overall health, our risk of illness, our mental health and happiness, and of course our weight. But as with eating, trends over the last fifty years are alarming, with more and more people leading sedentary lives. The numbers vary, but they're grim. According to the Centers for Disease Control, surveys suggest that only 20 percent of American adults say they meet the fitness guidelines for cardio and strength training, but the reality may be even worse. Researchers for the National Cancer Institute, who tracked people more precisely, using motion sensors, found that only 5 percent were getting at least thirty minutes of moderate-intensity activity most days of the week.

The gym is packed with new members in January who resolve to work out every day. This approach can be very motivating in the short term but usually isn't sustainable. Once again, it's the power-through-it approach, focused on external motivation and punishment/reward (think "no pain, no gain" and the glistening, unattainable bodies on display in running-shoe ads). For some, it's too intimidating to start, while many others begin and then fizzle out. And some people overdo exercise, which can be as harmful as under-doing it. All of these patterns are signs of the outside-in approach to change.

There's a balanced, middle way that starts with tuning in to yourself. As with eating, the *why* of exercise informs the *how*. Asking yourself, "What's my motivation to exercise? Who am I doing this for?" can yield important information. You might realize, for instance, that you've been jogging in order to keep up with (and maybe impress) your athletic sister-in-law, but you're actually not enjoying it—and what you really love is dancing. What if, instead of focusing on a narrow goal (losing a certain amount of weight or fitting into a certain dress) or viewing exercise as something you "should" do, you approached physical activity as an opportunity to support your total health (body and mind), gain energy, bring you pleasure and fun, and feel strong and competent? What if you did it for yourself alone?

Instead of focusing on the outcome—miles jogged, pounds lost, calories burned—you can focus on the process. That means tuning in to how your body is feeling before, during, and after exercise. That helps keep you flexible. If you realize that your shoulder is getting sore while swimming, you can stop before it becomes an injury—and perhaps vary your routine to include other activities. For most people, it helps to vary among a few activities, both to prevent injury and to stave off boredom. If you notice that you are resistant to the idea of exercising, remember *why* you're exercising—what you want in the long run. Rather than asking yourself, "Do I feel like exercising?" remind yourself why it's important to you.

When done in a balanced, mindful way, exercise becomes a positive feedback loop for a simple reason: it feels good! Even if you feel some discomfort or fatigue while you're exercising, you'll feel the benefits soon afterward. In fact, the benefits are often felt more quickly with exercise than with dietary changes. Our bodies and brains—everything from our blood vessels and mitochondria to our brain's feel-good neurotransmitters—function better when we're moving regularly. Finding your way to the right routine—not too little, not too much, and something you enjoy—is vital for self-care and total health.

Create Your Own Eating Culture

Just as creating your own exercise pattern is crucial, developing your own eating culture can also help to build your foundation. The word "diet" refers not only to a weight-loss plan but also to the foods, dishes, and eating styles associated with a traditional culture. In Italy, for instance, people have been eating fresh vegetables and herbs, fish, fresh pasta, olive oil, and small amounts of meat and cheese for centuries. In parts of Japan, rice, fish, seaweed, and vegetables are staples. In India, richly spiced vegetable and rice dishes prevail.

It's no coincidence that many cultures with long-standing traditional diets have lower rates of obesity and chronic illness than we see in the United States. Traditional diets consist of whole foods that are brimming with the nutrients our bodies need to thrive and resist disease. In cultures with a long culinary history, preparing wholesome foods is a natural focus in life. People aren't frantic about food the way many Americans tend to be. They prepare food slowly and eat slowly; they don't expect meals to be ready immediately, and they savor their meals. While many of these traditional diets are disappearing, overall, people who eat diets traditional to their culture tend to feel anchored and less confused about their choices—and therefore less likely to lapse into a diet mentality.

In the United States, a relatively new country of mixed heritage, there's no unifying anchor. While some Americans certainly grow up in a healthy eating environment (whether or not it's based on their family's heritage), many people feel adrift when it comes to eating. In a sense, conventional weight-loss diets and other extreme eating plans provide an anchor, a stand-in culture for people looking for advice on what and how to eat. But as we know, these plans tend to be neither healthy nor sustainable. And while losing weight is a healthy goal for a lot of people, doing so by eating packaged diet foods—many of which increase your risk of chronic illness—is a losing game.

Dangerous Diet Foods

It's not only the diet mentality that's damaging—it's the foods that often go along with it. The majority of diet foods—from soft drinks to packaged meals to "light" ice cream—are short on nutrition and long on unhealthy ingredients.

Like other processed foods, packaged diet foods often contain unhealthy fats, excessive amounts of sodium, chemical preservatives, and artificial colors and flavors. Some of them may also contain synthetic ingredients designed to reduce the fat or calorie content of foods. But substituting synthetic ingredients for natural ones comes at a price, as in synthetic fats like Olestra, which can cause digestive problems and reduce antioxidant absorption; artificial sweeteners such as acesulfame-K, which may disrupt thyroid function and has cancer-causing potential; and aspartame, which has been linked to cancer and neurological problems.

Diet soda deserves a special mention. Our consumption of it has more than doubled in the past thirty years. Diet sodas may be calorie-free, but studies suggest that drinking them long-term contributes to weight *gain*, not weight loss—and potentially an increased risk of diabetes. Initial research suggests that our brains don't register artificially sweetened beverages as satisfying, which may lead diet-soda drinkers to eat more sugary foods to quench their taste for sweetness. A recent population study also showed an association between consuming diet soda and a 44 percent increased risk of heart attacks and strokes.

Most healthy foods don't come in a package, certainly not one labeled "diet." You'll learn about the health benefits of whole foods (vegetables and fruits, lentils and beans, whole grains, nuts, fish and lean meats, herbs and spices) later in the book, but here's what's special about them for weight loss. Most whole foods, unlike packaged foods, have a healthy nutrients-to-calories ratio, and they're also generally harder to overeat than packaged foods (including flour-based products like bread, crackers, and pasta). The fiber and bulk of whole foods fill you up, and healthy sources of fat, such as avocados and nuts, are satisfying in small amounts.

Whatever kind of eating environment you grew up in, you can create *your own* eating culture—one that supports your health. As individuals and families, we can all work to develop healthy habits and rituals around food and eating.

You may already have an eating culture of sorts. You started to pinpoint it when you explored your eating rules/guidelines—or lack thereof—earlier in this chapter. Use the exercise below to go further and imagine your own optimal eating culture. Maybe you'd like to start shopping for vegetables every Saturday morning at the farmers' market, having friends over for Sunday night dinner, doing a prayer or centering practice before eating, joining the Meatless Monday campaign (see meatlessmonday.com), or taking twenty-five minutes to eat lunch at a table instead of eating quickly at your desk. Keep in mind that no culture is built in a day, and that instituting one small change at a time is more effective than trying to overhaul all your habits at once.

Exercise: Visualize Your Eating Culture

Jot down bullet points about the eating culture that you currently inhabit. What are your habits and rituals? Which of these support your health, and which do not? Next, spend ten minutes visualizing an alternative culture, with you as the kind of eater you'd like to be. What do you see yourself eating for breakfast? For lunch? For dinner? Who's with you during meals, and where are you? When and where do you shop for food? Who prepares it, and how and when? What is your role? Let your mind wander. When you're finished, write down your vision.

Goals for Sustainable Change

You've envisioned your best self and your ideal eating culture. You've explored your values and created healthy guidelines for yourself. And you've assessed your Wheel of Health to see what areas of your life are least satisfying and may be useful places to implement change. Now it's time to create goals that help you move forward on your journey in a sustainable way.

People are very familiar with goals but tend to approach them in one of two unhelpful ways: either they're vague or they're unrealistic. Vague goals are broad ideas about change with little specificity, such as "I'm going to eat better," "I'm going to get in shape," or "I'm going to start meditating." Vague goals lack guidance and often leave people without any idea of where to begin. Unrealistic goals, on the other hand, are impossible to achieve in a healthy way or don't take real life into account, such as "I'm going to lose 20 pounds in six weeks" or "I'm going to exercise for an hour every morning, before leaving for work at 7 A.M." Unrealistic goals set us up for the failure-shame-avoidance spiral that's at the heart of the diet paradigm.

The antidote to vague goals is specificity, and that includes time lines. Whereas "I'm going to get in shape" is vague and open-ended, "I'm going to speed-walk for twenty minutes, three days a week" is specific and time-bound. You need to know when you have met your goal; in the former you won't, but in the latter you will. So whether you're creating goals for eating, exercise, or the mindfulness practice you'll begin in the next chapter, ask yourself, "Is this goal time-bound?" and "Is this goal specific enough that it will be crystal clear when I have met it?"

Whatever behaviors you are trying to change, it is imperative to track them in either a written or electronic form. The research is quite clear; keeping data on your progress will help you stay accountable to yourself and support your success in changing behavior. Some people track their progress on goals in a simple journal like the one you have already started. Others benefit from specific formats such as the sample tracker we provide in chapter 5 for monitoring hunger and fullness and the one in chapter 7 for monitoring the thoughts, emotions, and events around eating. Still others use electronic apps that are available to track eating and exercise patterns. It is not important *how* you track, but *that* you track and evaluate your progress on goals regularly. The time lines of your goals will make it obvious when to evaluate your progress. For example, take the goal above of "speed-walking twenty minutes, three days per week." For this goal, the behavior to track is speed-walking, and specifically how long and how often you do it each week. The time to evaluate your progress is each week.

Your success is also linked to how carefully and realistically you set your goals—asking yourself, "Can I achieve this goal in a healthy way?

Can I make this fit into my life?" In addition, infusing your goals with some degree of flexibility can help you keep moving forward even when "life happens" and can help you resist all-or-nothing thinking. To that end, we often coach patients to create three tiers for a given goal—optimal, desirable, and minimal. Your **optimal goal** is the ideal you are striving for; it is probably not achievable on a regular basis right now. The **desirable goal** is one you feel you can achieve most of the time, given your life and circumstances. Your **minimal goal** is your backup plan, what you feel you can realistically do even when life throws you curveballs. Annie, a patient who ate mostly packaged, processed food and wanted to start cooking from scratch, came up with the following three-tiered goal:

Optimal goal:	Cook dinner from fresh ingredients six nights a week.
Desirable goal:	Cook dinner from fresh ingredients three nights a week—and make batches that will allow for leftovers.
Minimal goal:	Prepare a fresh salad or fresh cooked vegetables five nights a week.
Behavior to track:	Number of times I cook dinner from fresh ingredients per week, as well as number of times I prepare fresh salad or fresh cooked vegetables per week.

You can use this framework to create your own goals for any section of the Wheel of Health, including eating and exercise. Select one area from the Wheel of Health and create a set of goals for this week. Track your progress in writing and report it to a friend. You can also apply this system to your mindfulness practice, which you will begin in the next chapter.

Change from the Inside Out

Lasting weight loss and healthy habits are about the long game—making *sustainable* changes—which calls for a process that's diametrically opposed to dieting. Instead of fast and furious, this process is slow and steady. Instead of relying on outside authority, it relies on your own awareness, senses, knowledge, and wisdom. Instead of being punitive and rigid, it's compassionate and flexible—taking your whole self and your real life into account.

Marianne, age 55, had dieted off and on for decades—and saw herself as a failure for never sticking with a plan. In our program, she realized that her thought patterns and approach to change—not a lack of willpower—were keeping her trapped. "I used to be an all-or-nothing thinker," she explains. "If I couldn't do all of it, I wouldn't do any of it." So when she began a restrictive diet or ambitious exercise plan and found herself unable to follow it, she'd quit and berate herself. "You blew it again" was her constant refrain. Learning to identify her all-or-nothing thinking and creating goals for sustainable change were revolutionary. "Suddenly I realized that, hey, if I can't do sixty minutes of exercise, I can do fifteen. Or if I eat an unhealthy lunch, it's not 'game over'—I can get back on track at dinnertime."

A year into this shift, she has lost 15 pounds and feels great about herself. What's more, it has translated into the rest of her life. She says, "When I'm trying to solve a problem at work or at home, it's no longer all or nothing. Instead, I think, 'Okay, what *piece* of it *can* I do?'" For any given situation, there aren't just one or two options, and she no longer views herself as being either "on track" or a "failure." She feels a great deal more freedom and flexibility in her habits and in her life.

As you begin Part II of the program, you'll see that the awareness that's at the heart of sustainable change—the kind that Marianne developed—is not the result of a one-time revelation, but rather daily practice.

PART II

Building Your Foundation

CHAPTER 4

The Practice of Change

"At any moment, you have a choice that either leads
you closer to your spirit or further away from it."

—Thich Nhat Hanh

We all wish for positive change to come sweeping in like the wind, transforming us overnight. That's part of the diet fantasy: presto, change-o, you're different! But as with everything else in life, wishing doesn't make it so. Gaining insight into the internal and external forces that shape your eating habits and developing intrinsic motivation—in part by connecting to your values—are essential. But *actually changing* your behavior can remain discouragingly difficult—not because you're inherently lazy or self-destructive, but because eating is an automatic behavior you've been doing for decades.

In recent years, scientists have zeroed in on the neuroscience that creates habits and holds them in place. Doing an activity a certain way, again and again over time, gradually creates neural pathways in the brain so that the behavior becomes automatic, something we do without thinking. This process, known as procedural learning, occurs for mundane activities that most of us learn as children, such as brushing our teeth and tying our shoes, and it can occur for eating habits that we've come to follow almost automatically, whether they're healthy or unhealthy. It's helpful to think of any learned behavior that gets wired into our brains as a **packaged response.** Some packaged responses involve sections of the brain called reward centers, making them even more tenacious and complex. Smoking, gambling, drinking alcohol, and eating high-sugar-content or high-fat-content foods fall into this category.

To understand how packaged responses work, let's look at a common one that most of us can remember learning: driving. If you learned as a teenager, you probably still remember those herky-jerky first attempts that took all of your attention and focus, along with the look of thinly veiled terror on the face of your mom, dad, older sibling, or driving instructor sitting in the passenger seat. But over time, the separate, specialized skills that driving requires—steering, accelerating or braking, shifting gears—gradually merged into a smooth, cohesive whole. Driving became automatic, something that you do without thinking much about. After years of experience, it's now a packaged response.

Now imagine that tomorrow, someone instructs you to drive in a whole new way: to brake with your left foot (instead of your right foot) and steer with your knees (instead of your hands). And then you get in the car and struggle to follow those instructions, eventually reverting to the way you've been driving for years. Why? Driving means something very specific to your body and your brain—it's wired in your nervous system, and it can't be rewired through sheer force of will. But it *can* be relearned differently.

Like driving, eating habits, over time, get stored in our brains as packaged responses. From a health perspective, popping open a Coke every night when you get home or popping chips into your mouth while finishing projects at work are habits worth changing. But on a neurological level, following eating habits such as those are simply what your brain and body know how to do.

Packaged responses that involve eating are more complex than driving or tying your shoes, in that they involve many more chemicals—peptides, hormones, and neurotransmitters—throughout the body. Perhaps more important, whatever associations you learned between eating and emotions may also be packaged together: reaching for carbohydrates when you're upset, for instance, is a common packaged response. These packaged responses are often automatic, entrenched, and encoded into our brain physiology. These associations likely helped you cope in some way in the past. If done too often, though, the costs outweigh the benefits, and it might be time to build new associations.

Insights and Inspirations: Erika, age 47

Every night, I watch three hours of news while I'm cooking, eating, and drinking wine. It's delicious and comfortable. I've been doing it just about every night for years. It's definitely "automatic"— I walk from the garage to the kitchen and pour myself wine before even putting my purse down. At the end of the night, though, I usually feel sick because I've eaten too much, and I often feel like I've wasted three hours.

Rewiring the Brain

The good news is that our brains are "soft-wired," not hard-wired. They have neuroplasticity, meaning that they can be rewired, with new neural pathways. That's not a quick or easy process—it takes time, intention, and *practice*. To undo a packaged response like eating, and its associations, you need, first and foremost, a method for taking the package apart.

Enter mindfulness. A philosophy grounded in daily practice, mindfulness cultivates the attitude and the skills necessary to tease out the individual pieces of a packaged response like eating—and the tools to change it.

The skills that you'll learn in this book are a form of **applied mindfulness,** which blends ancient tradition and modern science. The essence of the practice—mindfulness meditation—originates from Buddhist teachings. At the University of Massachusetts Medical Center in the 1970s, Jon Kabat-Zinn, Ph.D., created a program that translated some of these teachings into a secular context, Mindfulness Based Stress Reduction (MBSR). MBSR was designed to help people cope with stress, pain, and a variety of acute and chronic illnesses. The dramatic success of MBSR—it's now taught at more than 200 health centers, and its benefits have been proven in multiple studies—gave rise to related forms of applied mindfulness, including the mindful-eating program you're learning here.

The heart of mindfulness practice is paying attention on purpose, with kindness and curiosity, to what you are experiencing in the present—in both your body and your mind. This might not sound like a big deal, but paying attention is the *opposite* of what both our external culture and our learned packaged responses encourage us to do (to stay unconscious) and the opposite of what most of us are used to doing. Practicing mindfulness has the power to interrupt automatic and reactive behavior—which for many people includes unhealthy eating. By practicing mindfulness, you begin to notice the subtle underlying thoughts, emotions, and physical sensations that drive your habits, and that awareness is the beginning of change.

When you tease apart an eating-related packaged response, you realize that there are some aspects of automatic behavior that you actually do have control over. You learn that what feels like a single event—overeating at lunch, for example—is actually a series of tiny "micro-events" all linked together. You might still be bombarded by the seductive smell of freshly baked muffins at the bakery on your way to your office, but you're able to pause before walking in, buying one, and wolfing it down; in that pause, you realize and experience the power to make a different choice. So paying attention, simple as it sounds, can be revolutionary.

Paying attention does not happen automatically, though. It takes intention and practice, in the form of daily meditation. You'll start that later in the chapter, and the exercise below, 20 Breaths (adapted from Michael Baime, M.D.), will get you started. It's the first in a series of **mindfulness tools**—useful practices that you can carry with you in your mental toolkit. Many people, especially those starting a meditation practice, find that being guided through meditation provides an additional anchor to help settle the mind. Throughout the book, when you see an audio symbol, it indicates you can find audio recordings of the exercises at www.dukeintegrativemedicine.org.

🔊 *Your Mindfulness Toolkit*

Here are the tools you'll add to your toolkit throughout the chapter. They'll form the foundation of your daily mindfulness practice. Once you've practiced them a lot, you can also use them when you feel overwhelmed or when you're slipping into unhealthy behaviors.

- 20 Breaths
- Mini-Meditation
- Daily Sitting Meditation
- Body Scan
- Loving-Kindness Meditation

As a preparation for meditation, 20 Breaths gives you practice paying attention in a new way: *disengaging* from the distractions in your mind while *focusing* on something new—your breathing. Wherever you are, whatever time it is, take five minutes to do this exercise.

🔊 Mindfulness Tool: 20 Breaths

In this exercise, think of each breath as a separate event. Each breath gives you the chance to practice focusing on something and to disengage your attention from whatever is distracting you. In order to fully notice the next breath, you have to disengage from whatever else is going on and fully focus on the count and experience of the breath itself.

1. Get settled in a comfortable seated position, and close your eyes.

2. Let your stomach expand and contract as you breathe in and out. As you breathe in, you can imagine there is a bal-

loon in your stomach expanding with the in-breath, allowing space around the organs in your core. As you breathe out, just let the air flow easily out of the balloon. You may want to place a hand on your abdominal area and experience this gentle rise and fall. While two or three deep breaths often help to relax at first, it is not necessary to take very deep breaths; rather, let your breath relax and come to its own natural rhythm.

3. Once you are settled, just say to yourself, silently, "Breathing in one," then "Breathing out one" for the first breath; then "Breathing in two . . . out two," etc. Go up to ten, then count backward, nine through zero.

What the Science Says: Mindfulness, Brain Changes, and Behavior

Making mindfulness meditation a routine part of your day has myriad benefits, many of which have been studied by behavioral scientists and neuroscientists. As you'll see, some of the following proven benefits are obviously linked to eating, and others are more subtly linked. All of them can help you change your eating habits. A mindfulness practice has been shown to help people:

- decrease habitual reactions to stressful situations
- reduce everyday anxiety
- recognize and fully experience emotions without being overwhelmed by them
- recognize information in the body (sensations)
- decrease the power of inner criticism and self-directed judgment
- recognize distorted thinking
- strengthen the part of the brain that processes positive emotions

- increase self-compassion and empathy for others
- increase the likelihood of making positive choices regarding behaviors, in particular, food choices
- improve immune system functioning
- reduce pain
- enhance working memory

Some of these changes are even seen in the brain. In one study of MBSR participants, MRI scans showed that after eight weeks of daily mindfulness meditation, brain areas related to memory, learning, and emotional regulation all increased in size. And in a study that showed a dramatic decrease in everyday anxiety among healthy people who were trained in mindfulness meditation, the regions of the brain that regulate thinking, emotion, and worrying—the anterior cingulate cortex and ventromedial prefrontal cortex—showed more activity in a way that suggests gaining more control of emotions.

Taking the Package Apart: Sensations, Thoughts, and Emotions

Undoing the packaged responses that aren't serving you well starts by tuning in to what's happening in your body and mind—specifically, physical sensations, thoughts, and emotions.

We're often "in our heads," rather than our bodies, but tuning in to our bodies yields very important information. Noticing your body's hunger and fullness signals and the way food really tastes, for instance, can radically alter your experience of eating. (You'll get to practice that in chapters 5 and 6.) Or you might notice that in the afternoons, after sitting at your desk all day, you feel a wave of fatigue and your shoulders start to ache—and that you tend to respond by going to the vending machine and buying M&Ms. Noticing sensations *as they're happening* allows you to respond in a healthy way, which can stop the domino effect that leads to unhealthy eating. When you feel that afternoon fatigue and pain, for instance, you can respond by taking a ten-minute walk outside instead of eating M&Ms.

Recognizing your thoughts may sound straightforward, but it's difficult for many people because we tend to *identify* with our thoughts instead of recognizing them for what they are: discrete mental "events" that contain information—information that may or may not be true and may or may not be helpful. Beliefs—thoughts that are so deeply ingrained that we hold them as truth—are especially tenacious. Suppose you eat a piece of cheesecake and just "know" that you did so because you have no self-control. That so-called knowledge is a belief, not a fact (and you might recognize its all-or-nothing nature from our discussion in the last chapter). It's important to know that we can be misled by our thoughts. When we believe that we should be a certain way, or that we need certain things, we're often expressing patterns or messages absorbed from others or our culture in general. Not only are these beliefs often false, they also do not serve us well. When you recognize a thought or belief, you can ask, *Do I know that to be true? How does that thought make me feel? How do I act on that thought?* Take, for example, a woman in the dressing room who just "knows" she should be a size 6. Where does this "knowledge" come from? What does that belief cause her to feel? How does she act on that belief?

During meditation, you'll practice noticing your thoughts. When you get good at that, you'll be able to notice your thoughts in your day-to-day life. And that gives you an opportunity to examine them, question their validity, and change the actions those thoughts inspire. In traditional mindfulness practice, people learn to observe thoughts as they form—and the thoughts then fade away without demanding a response. In *applied* mindfulness, if you determine a thought to be untrue or unhelpful, you can just watch the thought fade (as in traditional mindfulness)—or you can *change the thought* if it helps you to change your actions. Suppose, for example, that your office is piled high with paperwork. "My office is such a mess. I will never be able to clean it up," you think—and in response to that thought you go to get a snack (even though you're not hungry). When you recognize this pattern, you can intentionally examine and change your thought. The self-defeating thought, "I will never be able to clean it up," can become "I'm going to spend ten minutes organizing the papers on my desk."

As for emotions, we all experience them but don't always know how to identify them or what to do with them. Part of this is cultural. Compared with other societies, ours is very focused on problem-solving and *doing* (instead of being), and on thinking instead of feeling. We don't know what to *do* with emotions. And when emotions are welcomed, it is usually only the positive ones. The negative ones are messy, unpleasant, and irrational, and on our path to adulthood, most of us gain very little information or skills about how to manage them. Some emotions, such as sadness and anger, tend to be shied away from, devalued, and even punished from an early age. In some families and at school, children are told both explicitly and implicitly to "be nice," not to cry, not to be mad, and not to be scared.

Suppressing emotions in certain circumstances can mean they erupt in others. The flip side of denying emotions is being overwhelmed by them, which is also common. People sometimes get stuck in anger, snapping at their spouses and children; or in fear, imagining the most serious possible cause of mysterious physical symptoms. As with thoughts, we *overidentify* with feelings and can't see them for what they are. Many people respond to emotions—whether they're suppressed or overwhelming—with eating; you'll learn about these patterns in depth in chapter 7.

Mindfulness teaches a **middle road** to working with emotions, between the extremes of suppressing them and getting carried away by them. As with thoughts, it's possible to experience your feelings while maintaining a wedge of distance—we call this becoming the **Observer.** When you do that, you're able to see emotions for what they are—and learn from them.

Becoming aware of your inner world—sensations, thoughts, and emotions—through mindfulness can help you change your eating habits in a number of ways. The focus of this chapter is getting to know your own mind through meditation, which slows down the swirl of triggers that can lead to mind*less* eating and gets you in touch with a source of internal wisdom that we call your **Inner Compass.** This compass helps you make healthier choices about eating and exercise. Mindfulness can also be applied directly to the experience of eating, as with the woman in chapter 1 who eats her roasted fish, greens, and squash slowly and with great attention. You'll get to practice that in chapters 5 and 6. And finally, keeping in mind the connections between eating and other areas of life, illustrated in the Wheel of Health, practicing mindfulness can lead to lower stress and greater balance in your life, both of which support healthier eating habits.

Mindfulness Principle 1: Be Here Now

"Be here now," one of the mantras of mindfulness, might sound overly simplistic when you first hear it. Where else would you be? But when you start paying attention, you realize that while you're "here" physically, your mind is often busy burrowing into the past or projecting into the future. What's the problem with this? You end up reacting to the dramas that play out in your mind, which often have little or nothing to do with what's actually happening in the present moment. What's more, you *miss* a lot of what's happening in the present.

Think about it: how often have you been doing one thing—commuting to work, taking a shower, eating dinner with your family—and stressing about something that happened earlier in the day or worrying about what's going to happen tomorrow? But here's the key: more often than not, what's happening in the present moment is much more tolerable— even pleasant—than what's ahead of us or behind us. And even when the present moment is unpleasant, being aware of and present for it as the Observer rather than mentally running away from it can stave off a lot of suffering. You deal with events as they occur, and from a healthy distance.

Not being present can lead to myriad unhealthy eating patterns. Rather than contending with emotions like sadness and anger, some people overeat to "stuff" their feelings down. Not being present in our bodies means that we miss our bodies' hunger and fullness signals. These signals are the body's innate way of alerting you when to start and when to stop eating. Ignoring them is like driving on a busy road with no stop signs or traffic lights. Consider Samantha, age 36, who worked as a communications coordinator at a nonprofit and got into the habit of eating lunch at her desk while reading through emails. Generally, she ate very little, nibbling half a sandwich or an apple and a few pieces of cheese. Sometimes she forgot to eat entirely. It's not that she wasn't hungry, but she was too stressed and "in her head" to notice what was going on in her body. By the time she picked up her daughter from day care and arrived home, however, she was so ravenous that she ate whatever she could get her hands on—sometimes half a bag of potato chips or a big handful of Oreos. When she sat down to dinner with her family—usually a healthy meal that she had prepared—she often was too full to eat much and had a stomachache.

How can being present shift your eating habits? If you tend to overeat or eat unhealthy food in response to stress, remaining in the present allows you to relax, mentally and physically, and stop the reactive cycle that leads to overeating (or choosing high-sugar or high-fat foods). Being present also keeps you in touch with what's happening in your body—notably, signals of hunger and fullness that are very easy to ignore when your mind is going a mile a minute, as in Samantha's story. And finally, when you're present, you can consciously direct your attention to your sensory experience while you're eating, noticing the textures, tastes, and smells that you might usually miss because you're distracted or eating quickly. Fully engaging your senses will help you better enjoy smaller amounts of food.

What the Science Says: Mindful Eating and Health

Behavioral scientists and health professionals know that changing eating habits and losing weight are notoriously difficult. This is largely because most approaches don't get to the heart of the problem—the myriad reasons *why* people are eating the way they do—or equip people with realistic strategies. In a program of NIH-funded clinical trials begun by Jean Kristeller, Ph.D., and in one industry trial that tested our mindfulness-based approach, study participants decreased compulsive eating habits, improved self-control with regard to eating, lost weight at a gradual and sustainable pace, maintained significant weight loss for at least sixteen months, and improved a number of indices of well-being, including reduced depression, lower perceived stress, and greater self-esteem. A remarkable 55 percent of those in the mindful-eating program who had metabolic syndrome (a collection of conditions that can lead to diabetes and heart disease) reversed this condition.

Taming the Monkey Mind

Our minds have a tendency to zigzag wildly through time and space, through fears, hopes, and frustrations. This is not a new development. What's come to be known as "monkey mind"—the voices in our heads that constantly chatter, screech, and carry on—is at best distracting static and at worst a reactive cycle that leads to unhealthy patterns, including overeating and eating unhealthy food.

Being in the "here and now" doesn't just happen—it takes practice. And while this has always been true, we're now living in a society that is essentially monkey mind writ large. Almost everything about our culture brings us somewhere else. The media we consume—both news and entertainment—takes us out of the present, whether we're watching heart-wrenching events unfold on the news or TV shows in which we inhabit an imaginary world. Advertising bombards us from all angles, and its fundamental mission is to take us out of the present and into a future fantasy with whatever's being sold. Whether we're online or watching TV, we can, in a matter of seconds, daydream about a dozen things: the feel of heated seats on a new SUV in the winter; enjoying the silky, shiny locks promised by that hair-dye ad; experiencing the bliss of walking along a tranquil beach at sunset, mojito in hand. The Internet, which most Americans have at their fingertips, is a 24/7 portal for escaping the here and now.

Our emotions can also take us out of the present. Consider Aimee, age 41, who was feeling preoccupied and anxious about an upcoming visit from her older sister, Jenny, who had been distant and critical of Aimee when they were growing up. Aimee began losing sleep worrying about what Jenny would think of her house, her circle of friends, even her cooking, and about how they would get along once they were under the same roof again. Aimee ended up feeling distracted and unproductive at work from lack of sleep. Too tired to plan, much less cook, a healthy meal one night, she ate a frozen chicken potpie followed by a large bowl of ice cream. Her eating habits devolved from there. Two days before the visit, Jenny called to say she had to cancel the trip—her son had the flu—and sounded genuinely sorry. Aimee was left feeling ridiculous for getting herself so stressed out over nothing and at a loss for how to get her eating habits back on track.

We've all been in a situation like Aimee's—getting worked up over a perceived threat that never comes to pass. But even if her sister had come, and even if it was a difficult visit, the time Aimee spent dwelling on it *before it was even happening* created a lot of unnecessary suffering— including sending her eating habits into a tailspin.

Aimee's story shows how unexamined thoughts and emotions, along with high stress, can lead to unhealthy eating, whether that means over-eating, forgetting to eat, or opting for unhealthy food. Learning mindfulness helps to keep you in the present, which makes you less prone to reactive eating; instead of having your awareness consumed with worries about what might happen (as in Aimee's case) or what already happened, you can focus on what is happening now. Practicing mindfulness can also let you "course correct," so that one unhealthy eating incident doesn't spiral into a pattern.

Focusing on the here and now requires skills and practice. You'll learn a number of techniques, but the most important one is daily meditation. You'll be building your meditation practice throughout this chapter, and it will serve as a cornerstone of our program. So let's start practicing. Take five minutes to do the following Mini-Meditation.

🔊 Mindfulness Tool: Mini-Meditation

1. Set a timer for five minutes, and sit comfortably with a straight spine. Close your eyes gently and breathe normally, just letting the air flow in and out at its own pace. Notice what your breath feels like as you inhale and exhale.

2. Notice what's happening in your body and your mind. Do you notice sensations? Thoughts? Emotions? Observe them, and then refocus on the breath, using it as an anchor that you return to.

3. When the timer rings, open your eyes.

If you're like most people, you might be worried that you "did it wrong" or you're "just not cut out for meditating" because your mind flitted here, there, and everywhere for what felt like the entire time. That's monkey mind in action—perfectly normal. The point of mindfulness meditation isn't to relax or empty your mind of all thoughts; it's to gain awareness of what's happening in your mind and body. When you *notice* your thoughts instead of getting caught up in them, you're creating a space that wasn't there before. This space holds the key to change. As you develop your practice, you'll see this in action. By practicing daily meditation, your awareness will begin to carry over into your day-to-day life.

As you learn more about mindfulness, you'll expand your meditation practice. But if you put the book down for a couple of days or feel like the longer exercises are too demanding for you at the moment, do either 20 Breaths or the Mini-Meditation three times every day. Bring awareness of your mind's meanderings—and how they diverge from what is happening in the present—to your everyday activities, too. It doesn't happen overnight, but you'll be surprised at how powerful both having the *intention* to be present and *practicing* presence can be. Here's what some of our program participants started realizing when they paid attention to the present:

- Marianna, 47, who had a habit of eating in response to stress: *I'd be worried about next month's travel or yesterday's tension with my mother-in-law, but right here, right now, everything is okay.*
- Jennifer, age 32, who had never had an exercise routine: *I'm wrapped up in fantasies about redoing our kitchen, but right here, right now, I realize my body's stiff from sitting all day, and I could use a walk, instead of looking at design blogs online.*
- Greg, age 56, who always ate lunch at the same sub shop: *I'd generally just walk there automatically and always order the same thing: a large meatball sub. When I started paying attention, I noticed a little Middle Eastern place on the corner with delicious food—much healthier, lots of veggies. I also noticed how much better it made me feel than my usual lunch.*

As you practice these short meditations, begin to notice what your body and mind are up to—both while meditating and in your day-to-day life. You might notice, for instance, that it takes longer than five minutes to focus your attention on the here and now. In terms of eating, you might notice that you start buzzing with anxiety when you're trying to finish a work project and consequently "forget" to eat—and then get so hungry that you scarf down a candy bar from the vending machine. Or you might notice that the transition from work to home is a big stressor: instead of the quiet time you are craving after a busy day, there's dinner to be made and homework to help with—and if you haven't eaten since lunchtime, you may be shaky from low blood sugar and prone to eating unhealthy snacks. You are just noticing your internal world—body sensations, thoughts, and emotions. Jot down your observations in your journal.

Mindfulness Principle 2: Stop Judging

Our minds are talented, tireless storytellers. Even more than making simple observations, we constantly spin tales and make judgments—about the world, other people, and ourselves. When we see a coworker duck into her office looking tired, we create a story about why. While reading a neighborhood LISTSERV post about a political issue, we make a judgment that the neighbor is a "good" or "bad" person. When we don't hear back about a job we've applied for, we assume it's because we flubbed the interview (even though we felt great afterward). When we see a child misbehaving at the grocery store, we quietly judge the parents.

For people who struggle with eating habits and weight, judgment plays a powerful role. We often react to simple facts with powerful condemnation about ourselves. "I ate a whole bowl of ice cream" (a fact) gets turned into "I have no willpower and am going to be overweight all my life!" (a judgment). "My stomach has gotten bigger in the last year" (a fact) becomes "I'm a fat slob" (a judgment). These judgments are the voice of the Inner Critic. In chapter 3 we discussed some of the ways that the Inner Critic undermines change—it takes up a great deal of space in our mind, takes us on an emotional roller coaster, and makes us reluctant to see reality. This happens so quickly, though, that it can feel out of our control, almost as if the mind can't help itself. The voice of the Inner Critic becomes automatic because it gets repeated over and over, usually without our realizing it.

With practice, you can learn to simply observe. Intentionally withholding judgment, or **non-judgment,** is another principle of mindfulness. Instead of criticizing, praising, or otherwise judging, you simply observe "what is." Non-judgment allows you to parse the facts of a situation, or the data, from the story your mind spins about it; it slows down the cascade of thoughts and emotions and creates a space to simply take note. Rather than descending into the consuming and counterproductive failure-shame-avoidance spiral, practicing non-judgment frees you to notice *more*. And the more we notice, the more options we have to respond. Take Justine, age 62, who tends to overeat at night, feel ashamed afterward, and then zone out in front of the TV to distract herself from the emotional and physical discomfort she experiences. By practicing non-judgment, she might simply notice the discomfort in her over-full stomach. By acknowledging it without criticism or guilt, she allows herself the space to think about self-care. Instead of tuning out, she might respond by asking herself, "What would help my stomach feel better? A cup of peppermint tea? A brisk walk around the block?" Just posing those questions—which amount to "How can I take care of myself in a healthy way right now?"—is a radical shift from her previous pattern.

You might be thinking, "But she still overate in front of the television!" and that non-judgment sounds like an excuse to let yourself off the hook. But interrupting the failure-shame-avoidance spiral does *not* amount to letting yourself off the hook. To the contrary, objective awareness begets more awareness—and that allows for accountability. Further, when you start practicing non-judgment, it eventually will help you shift course *before* (or while) engaging in unhealthy eating habits. So maybe the next time Justine sits down to eat at night, she'll be aware of her pattern and make a different choice about how much she eats.

Insights and Inspirations: Lessley, age 44

For years, I overate—and every time, I berated myself for having no control. When I was finally able to stop beating myself up for eating too much, I was able to see the pattern of my habits: whenever I felt the slightest touch of hunger, I would start to feel really anxious. It was almost primal, as if I was scared I was going to starve! I felt like I had to eat immediately. By learning how to separate out the data (I'm starting to feel hungry) from the story (I need to eat now or something terrible will happen!), I've been able to cut down on overeating and relax more, too. But it was only possible when I stopped criticizing myself.

Exercise: Data versus Story

Teasing apart the data and the stories in your mind takes practice. Read the following examples and come up with healthy responses to the data. Then think of a couple of examples from your own life and habits.

1. Jumbled reaction: *I have a stomachache and I feel so disgusting after eating all that cookie dough. I wasn't even hungry; it just tasted so good. God, I have no willpower!*

   Story: *I'm disgusting; I have no willpower.*

   Data: *I ate cookie dough when I wasn't really hungry, and now my stomach hurts.*

   Healthy response to data: _____

   _____

2. Jumbled reaction: *My pants from last summer don't fit. I'm going to keep gaining and gaining until I'm obese like everyone else in my family. I'm so pathetic.*

   Story: *I'm pathetic; I'm destined to be obese.*

   Data: *I've gained weight, and my pants don't fit.*

   Healthy response to data: _____

   _____

Now fill in a couple of examples from your own life related to your eating habits or your weight:

3. Jumbled reaction: _____

   _____

   Story: _____

   _____

Data: _____

_____

Healthy response to data: _____

_____

4. Jumbled reaction: _____

_____

Story: _____

_____

Data: _____

_____

Healthy response to data: _____

_____

Exercise: Non-judgment Days

For three days, keep your journal with you as you go through your day. Pay attention to your thoughts and jot down your negative judgments, especially those related to food, eating, or your body. Try to capture at least four examples. At the end of the three days, review them. For each, can you separate the data from the story? Write these down. For the *next* three days, do the same thing, but try to catch yourself in the moment when you're making a judgment and replace it with an objective observation—the data. Do you notice a difference in the way you feel or behave? It might feel unnatural, but over time, you will begin to more easily separate the data from the story. Daily meditation will help you with this. Remember, you're retraining your brain.

What About the Good Stories?

What about the "good" judgments, the times when we congratulate ourselves for sticking with our eating plan, losing weight, or looking great in new clothes? This is an area where applied mindfulness diverges from the tradition it hails from. The "grandmother" of mindfulness, Buddhism, teaches extreme neutrality, in which we dismantle the positive stories we tell about ourselves and the world along with the negative ones. If you praise yourself for having completed a 5K road race, traditional mindfulness would have you question that praise in much the same way that you would question self-criticism for not completing the race.

In applied mindfulness, we are helping people to achieve their health goals, and what matters to us is what works. We've found through studies and clinical practice that focusing on the positive, instead of extreme neutrality, can be very helpful. However, it can be delusional, too; focusing on feeling good about last night's healthy dinner while you're wolfing down a burger and chips for lunch doesn't make much sense. What matters, we've found, is *whether the judgment/story is helping you move toward your health goals.* So when you're feeling good about something eating- or exercise-related, simply ask yourself, "Is this helping me move toward my goals?" If it is, great! If it's not, don't pile on negative judgment. Return to the objective place of non-judgment and gather more data.

"Good story" examples

1. Jumbled reaction: *I ate a healthy lunch. I am really on a roll now!*

   Data: *I ate a healthy lunch.*

   Story: *I'm on a roll now.*

   Is the story helping me move toward my goal? How? *Yes. One healthy lunch isn't exactly being "on a roll," but feeling enthusiastic and confident gives me momentum to stay on track with my eating plan.*

What now? *Harness the positive energy and plan some healthy meals for the week. Maintain awareness of both my choices and my thoughts about those choices.*

2. Jumbled reaction: *It's okay that I've eaten fast food and sweets all weekend—I did well all week! I deserve it.*

   Data: *I ate well all week but have fallen back into my automatic habits this weekend.*

   Story: *The fact that I ate well this week means that it's okay to slide back into my automatic-eating patterns all weekend.*

   Is the story helping me move toward my goal? How? *No. I've been working to change my eating habits, and mindlessly sliding back into them reinforces them and makes it harder to get back on track.*

   What now? *I'm going to pay attention to my body and my mind to try to notice what sensations and thoughts set me on the path toward fast food and sweets. Next weekend, I'll come up with a plan that lets me stick to my eating guidelines and plan for some healthy indulgence, like a massage.*

Mindfulness Principle 3: Flex Your Kindness Muscle

Another principle of mindfulness, kindness, takes non-judgment a step further. Along with objectively observing your body's sensations, your thoughts and feelings, and your eating behaviors—seeing reality for what it is—it's possible to cultivate *active* compassion and kindness. When a baby is learning to walk, stumbles and falls are part of the learning process—and parents instinctively respond with love and encouragement. Changing the way you relate to food and your body is also very difficult and is not a linear process. As such, this learning calls for not only a nonjudgmental attitude, but a nurturing one. Compassion gets you a lot further than punishment. Like non-judgment, kindness frees you to notice more, and it also actively encourages positive change and growth. We see this again and again in our clinic, and scientific studies support this finding. A study of eighty-four women at Wake Forest University, for example, showed that increasing self-compassion could influence eating habits for the better.

Why is kindness so difficult? Here in the West, we prioritize "finding the problem," critical thinking, and focusing on what needs to be fixed. This plays out well in some contexts. We'd want our brain surgeon to be thinking critically and analyzing. In other contexts, such as learning new behaviors, it's counterproductive. Many of us direct love and kindness outward to our families and friends, but not inward toward ourselves. And for women in particular, relating compassionately to our bodies in all their "imperfection" is a 180-degree shift from what we're used to doing and what our culture teaches us to do. (More on this in chapter 8.) When it comes to food, we fear that kindness is tantamount to "anything goes." But the opposite is true. When we treat ourselves with true compassion, we *want* to take good care of our bodies.

Think of it this way: if you're feeling upset or disappointed about something, would you rather talk to a belittling tyrant (the Inner Critic) or a compassionate, caring friend who is interested in helping you change? Who would be more helpful? The answer is easy. In order to learn new behaviors, we need to be that compassionate friend *to ourselves*. Most of us wouldn't put up with character assassination from someone else, but that's exactly what we do to ourselves when we're having a hard time making changes. As with the first two mindfulness principles we discussed—being present and non-judgment—cultivating compassion is a practice. A mindfulness tool called Loving-Kindness Meditation, below, can get you started.

🔊 Mindfulness Tool: Loving-Kindness Meditation

1. Sit comfortably in a chair or on a cushion in a quiet place. With your eyes closed or, if you prefer, open but with a soft downward gaze, relax, and breathe easily and comfortably. Feel your energy settle in your body, effortlessly resting.

2. Begin to pull your awareness into your heart area, and let your breathing arise from that area. Think of the face of a special child, a pet, or someone very dear to you from whom you've felt great love. Imagine that face and sense the connection. Let that loving, warm feeling spread from your heart center throughout your chest. Savor that feeling. Then let it spread a little farther, through your torso and into your back. Gradually, over multiple gentle breaths, allow the warmth to spread throughout your entire body.

3. In your mind, repeat a four-part mantra, *May I be safe, may I be happy, may I be healthy, may I be kind.* If other adjectives or phrases speak more clearly to what you wish most deeply for yourself, feel free to use different ones in your four-part mantra (examples: *May I be joyful, May I be peaceful, May I be loving, May I be healed, May I live with ease, May I live life beyond fear*). Repeat the mantra until you feel a sense of well-being.

4. Now, visualize the circle of well-being you've created radiating outward to someone you love, such as a family member or close friend. Use this person's name in the mantra: for example, "May Emma be safe, may she be happy, may she be healthy, may she live with ease."

5. Continue radiating this message of well-being out to people you care about, one at a time, and then move on to acquaintances. You can also move the circle outward to those you don't know—specific people, or the people of your town, your state, your country, or the entire world.

6. Bring the practice to a conclusion when you feel complete with it, or when your practice time is up.

Insights and Inspirations: Kyre, age 46

I'm a teacher and a mother of three kids under 10, so I'm always busy and tending to someone. I'm not complaining; I have a lot to give and it comes naturally. But a few years ago, I got to a point where I was about 50 pounds overweight and just really out of shape. And in my mind, I criticized myself constantly for it—really mean stuff, things I'd never say to a student or my children. I didn't stop and think about what I was doing to myself at all, that all those insults really had power. Starting the mindfulness program made me stop and look at those thoughts and realize how uncaring they were. What was that about? The regular meditation and loving-kindness exercises let me see my patterns more clearly than I ever had and start to really take care of myself. If you tell yourself something enough times—bad or good—you start to believe it.

Putting It Together: A Daily Practice

The most important step in changing your relationship with food doesn't directly involve food at all—it involves sitting to meditate on a daily basis. Reading about mindfulness can give you insight, and quick exercises can help you relax, but reaping the benefits of mindfulness takes practice. To get to know your own mind, you have to spend some time with it.

Keeping in mind the three principles of mindfulness we've introduced—being in the present, non-judgment, and kindness—start meditating for fifteen minutes most days of the week. Use the instructions below—an expanded version of the Mini-Meditation. Every two weeks, increase your time by five minutes, aiming for a meditation time of twenty-five to thirty minutes. Patients often ask what the best time of day to meditate is, and the answer is, whenever you will do it! Many people find morning works best, while some prefer to do it right after work, and others at night. Pick a time of day when you can realistically set aside a half hour in a quiet space, and schedule it in your calendar as you would an appointment or a meeting.

Don't be surprised if you find meditating very uncomfortable or even boring. We're a very task-oriented society, focused on productivity and multitasking, on *doing* rather than *being*, often at the expense of our health. You're not going to instantly shed these cultural values, so at first you might find that meditation feels like a waste of time. As Shannon, age 33, summed up her experience doing guided meditation for the first time: "Our life is built on doing things, and my honest reaction was, 'This is silly, sitting here with my eyes closed listening to myself breathe.'" In one of our mindful-eating groups, a participant described learning to meditate like this: "It felt bizarre at first. It's as if someone said, 'Hey, put some peanut butter on the end of your nose.' I thought it was crazy. But I looked around at all the others with their eyes closed and decided that if everyone else can try, I can, too. I won't learn something new without trying. And I'm so glad I did." If you feel that way at first, notice those thoughts and feelings, but stick with the practice. You might even try to tease out, "What is the data, and what is my story?"

Remember, your current patterns are a product of years of conditioning. We do what we know how to do—and when you try to change your patterns, some aspects of you may protest. Just notice that. You might find that you have an aversion to being still and find a thousand things to do instead of meditate (clean your house, balance your checkbook, call a friend, watch a "very important" TV show, eat lunch, go shopping—the list can go on and on). Just notice that, too. Noticing your resistance is part of your practice.

Insights and Inspirations: Audrey, age 40

I've always felt a strong need to be occupied. With meditation, you really have to be with yourself. That can be a little bit scary. It gets better once you start doing it, but I still sometimes feel like I'd rather be doing something else—anything else. If I can breathe through that feeling, I can sink into the meditation and learn about my mind. I can learn how my behavior comes about.

🔊 Mindfulness Tool: Daily Sitting Meditation

Start by meditating for fifteen minutes each day. Every two weeks, increase your practice time by five minutes until you're practicing for at least twenty-five minutes.

1. Find a quiet and comfortable place. Set a timer for the amount of time you've decided to meditate (preferably one with a soft ring). Sit in a chair with both feet on the floor, or cross-legged on the floor if that's comfortable. (While yogis may sit in lotus position or other postures, that's not necessary for the practices in this book.) Either way, hold your head, neck, and back straight but not stiff. You want to convey to your mind, "I'm relaxed but alert."

2. Begin by focusing on your breathing, focusing on the sensation of air moving in and out of your body as you breathe. Feel your belly rise and fall; feel the air enter your nostrils and leave your body. Pay attention to the way each breath changes and is different. You may want to start with the 20 Breaths practice to give you some structure.

3. As you continue to focus on your breath, you may notice that thoughts or emotions arise. When thoughts come up in your mind, don't ignore or suppress them but simply notice them, remain calm, and then return your attention to your breathing. You might imagine thoughts as leaves floating down a river and imagine that you are sitting on the bank, watching the leaves (aka the thoughts) float by. During your practice, if you realize you are *in* the river, wrestling with the thoughts themselves, just climb back up the bank, settle, and observe them floating on by, using your breath to anchor you. The breath is your point of focus and refocus when your attention has wandered.

4. If an emotion comes up, just watch it. See if you notice whether it takes a certain course; often emotions rise and then fall. Can you take the Observer stance, letting your-

self feel but maintaining a certain distance that lets you see what's happening?

5. When you find that your mind wanders off, simply return to your breathing, without judgment. Remember not to be hard on yourself if this happens. You are just training your mind to be here now. Also notice any physical sensations that come up, with kindness and without judgment.

6. As the time comes to a close, take a moment to offer gratitude to yourself for taking this time for self-care, for creating this opportunity for yourself to settle and to learn. Get up gradually.

Insights and Inspirations: Siobhan, age 51

Meditating was a whole new thing for me. My mind is always churning; my train of thought always runs away from me. But the whole point is to be in the moment—to just experience this moment. And if you have a thought that comes into your mind, that's okay, just come back to where you are in that moment. I didn't think I'd be able to do it because of how crazy my brain is. But I could; I can. And I really get a lot out of it.

Setting Goals for Meditation

The benefits of meditation are cumulative, the result of regular practice. As with any new habit you're trying to forge, it's helpful to create goals for behavior you can sustain. Keeping in mind the importance of specificity, write down a three-tiered goal for your meditation practice here or in your journal, and note the behavior you'll track. Consider details such as what time of day you'll meditate, where you'll meditate, how long you'll meditate, and how frequently you'll meditate.

Optimal goal:

_____

Desirable goal:

_____

Minimal goal:

_____

Behavior to track:

_____

Understanding the Layers of Your Mind

Being "stuck in our heads," as most of us are, doesn't mean we understand our minds. Day to day, our thoughts and feelings shift quickly, as does the busy world we inhabit. It's hard to keep up with our minds' inner workings in the most basic sense, let alone analyze and understand them. But as you develop your mindfulness practice, you'll notice different aspects of your mind. Like muddy water that gently settles, your mind slows down and becomes more transparent, allowing you to access your inner wisdom. With more practice, your observational skills improve. These skills will help you as you learn to understand your thinking process and, more important, to relate to yourself in a kinder and wiser manner. And then you can examine and understand your mind—which helps you examine and better understand your eating habits, your health, and your life.

The model below—adapted from one created by our colleague, psychotherapist and meditation teacher Sasha Loring, M.Ed., L.C.S.W.—shows the mind with three distinct layers. If you started meditating only recently, don't be discouraged if you haven't experienced all these layers of mind. Remember the muddy water metaphor—clarity takes time. As you practice, see whether this model resonates for you and what kind of information each layer offers.

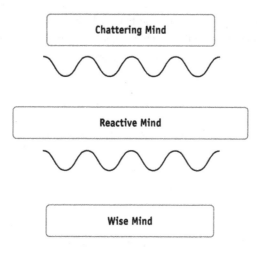

Chattering mind. The top, most accessible layer, also known as the "monkey mind," is made up of the constant stream of thoughts and judgments that can be difficult to settle.

Reactive mind. The second, deeper layer of mind is made up of the thoughts, beliefs, sensations, and emotions that tend to drive our behavior. These thoughts and emotions (which are usually the product of beliefs) often put up a screen, clouding our view of what actually *is*.

Wise mind. The deepest layer of mind is your wisest self. Here lies the inherent wisdom shared by all people, which is usually covered over with the chattering mind and the reactive mind. Our wisest selves can be accessed only when the other two layers are seen clearly for what they are and quieted down. With regular meditation practice, you can quiet the busy mind and access your wisest self.

Your Inner Compass

Think of your wise mind as your **Inner Compass,** an internal guide that has your best interest at heart. Following your Inner Compass gives you a sense of direction that helps you behave in healthier ways that align with what you most care about; it helps you live according to your values. We've found that using the Inner Compass helps people stay on track with good eating habits and find healthy balance in life. Your Inner Compass is at the heart of intrinsic motivation—as opposed to motivation based on ideas about what you "should" or "must" do.

Just as an actual compass helps you navigate a landscape, the Inner Compass helps you navigate your life and serves as a guide for the dozens of choices you face every day—*Do I go for a walk or sit and watch the news? Do I order the Greek salad with chicken or the "loaded" baked potato?* As you develop your meditation practice, you will be cultivating access to your Inner Compass. Practice distinguishing it from the other forces in your mind—the Inner Critic, the impulsive ego that "wants what it wants, now!," and the voices that tell you what you "should" do for some unclear reason. Connecting with your Inner Compass will help you feel calm and clear, rather than impulsive or chastened.

Exercise: Connecting to Your Inner Compass

After your meditation practice, spend five or ten minutes thinking and writing about your Inner Compass. Think of a time when you felt an inner voice directing you in a self-caring way, whether or not you acted on the voice. It could be an eating-related example or something else entirely. What did the inner wise voice say? How did it make you feel? If you've never experienced such a voice, imagine what it would say. How would it feel to be connected to such a voice on a regular basis? Do you have a sense of how your eating and exercise habits would be different? How your life might change? Are you willing to do the practice to gain that connection?

Coming Back to Sensation

Exploring our minds is central to mindfulness practice, but connecting with our physical selves is equally important. We are "living in our heads" so much of the time that it's easy to ignore or not even notice what our bodies are trying to tell us. People who struggle with weight, in particular, often shut off their awareness from their bodies out of fear, anxiety, or distress over how they think their body looks or what their physical limitations might be.

One excellent way to tune in to your mind and body is through a technique we call the **Body Scan**—a mindfulness tool that involves sequentially focusing on different areas of the body in order to notice the signals it may be sending you. The Body Scan is designed to help us "be" in the body, to feel what's happening moment to moment, which is different from *thinking about* the body.

🔊 Mindfulness Tool: Body Scan

1. Get comfortable in your chair, with your feet flat on the floor. Close your eyes or find a spot on the ground to softly focus on. Bring your attention to your breathing. Breathe in space to discover and accept what is. Breathe out tension, breathe in calm.

2. Take a few moments to feel your body as a whole, from head to toe. Feel the sensations associated with each part of your body. Then bring your attention to your feet. Direct your breathing to them, so that it feels as if you are breathing in through your feet and out from your feet. Allow yourself to feel any and all sensations from your feet. If you do not feel anything, let yourself become aware of that, too.

3. Now move on to your calves. Allow yourself to become aware of whatever sensations are present. With your attention focused on them, direct your breathing to them, so that

it feels as if you are breathing in through your feet, up your lower legs and calves, dwelling on the sensations of your lower legs. Breathe into that space and out from that space.

4. As you breathe in, now scan up your legs through your knees to your thighs. Allow yourself to become aware of whatever sensations are present, or not present. Direct your breathing to this area. If you find that you are thinking about, rather than experiencing, sensations in your thigh area, see if you can just notice the thoughts, but redirect your attention to the sensations.

5. Now progress upward to your genital area, buttocks, and hips. Allow yourself to become aware of any sensations that are present in these areas. Then breathe in through these areas—and out.

6. Move your attention all the way up to your lower back and stomach area. Dwell here for several breaths. What sensations do you experience? Are there areas in which you don't have sensation? Breathe in, letting yourself be aware of this area of your body. And breathe out.

7. Move your scan up to your lungs and your chest. Again, as you breathe in, attend to your lungs and chest, and the sensations you experience in these areas. As you breathe out, notice how the sensations change.

8. Now move up to your shoulders and down the arms. As you breathe in, attend to your shoulders, arms, and even hands—then breathe out.

9. Now scan your neck and face, allowing yourself to notice any sensations that you may be feeling in these areas. As you breathe in, attend to your neck, jaw, eyes, and forehead—then breathe out.

10. Take a few moments to feel your body as a "whole," from your toes up to your head. As you breathe in, attend to your whole body. As you breathe out, keep noticing.

11. Whenever you're ready, open your eyes.

Looking Within for Guidance

People experience remarkable shifts—sometimes subtle and sometimes dramatic—when they begin to practice mindfulness. Laney, age 41, who had been trying to change her eating habits for decades, had tried a number of diet programs. She'd follow a program to the letter, lose some weight, and when it was over, start overeating almost immediately. When she started doing our program, she realized that in the past, all of her energy was focused outward—on following the diet's instructions and pleasing the instructors. "I thought I could set new habits by following the program, but it never worked," she said. Looking within herself had never occurred to her. In one diet program she had attended, instructors graded their food diaries. "I was always oriented toward making the program's leaders happy. If I was deciding between yogurt or a candy bar, I'd choose the yogurt—because that's what they'd rather have me do," she said. "I never internalized any of the changes I made."

When Laney began to practice looking within, through meditation, it was a revelation. She said, "If you had told me that I could change my eating habits by being still and meditating every day, I would have laughed. It would have seemed ridiculous." She realized, though, that the twenty minutes she committed to being still were more powerful than any dieting program. She learned to identify her thoughts and emotions, and got in touch with her Inner Compass. "I didn't know I had that in me. I really didn't. Now when I choose the yogurt, or the salad, or the walk, it's me making a better choice for *me*—not someone else. And guess what? I make those better choices most of the time now."

You might not realize it now—you might not believe it—but both your mind and your body are treasure troves of wisdom. Learning certain practical skills and information is essential, too—knowing which foods help you stay healthy and understanding portion sizes, for example—and you will learn all of that. But in trying to change your habits, the most important skill by far is intentionally turning inward, being still, and getting to know your own mind and body. The information and wisdom you'll gather from these valuable sources trumps all others. But remember that mindfulness isn't magic; it's practice.

CHAPTER 5

The Goldilocks Principle

"Enough is as good as a feast."

—Proverb

Hunger is a primal sensation. The trigger that prompts us to seek out food is key to the functioning and health of our bodies and brains—our very survival.

We all know what hunger feels like, right? Yes . . . and no. As with other ancient instincts, the sensation of hunger has gotten complicated for many people in the modern world. Many clients who come to our clinic can easily recognize extreme hunger, but they have trouble sensing its subtler versions. Other people have the opposite pattern—they're hypersensitive to hunger and end up reaching for food at the slightest pang, or even at the thought that they *might* be hungry.

In addition to why we *start* eating—and whether or not this aligns with our physical hunger—there's the issue of when and why we *stop* eating. Overeating has become the norm in this country. While the body gives us cues about when it's had enough food, we often miss or ignore them. Many people wait until they're stuffed to stop eating or they eat too quickly, which doesn't give the brain time to register that the body has had enough.

Why is there such a disconnect between our eating patterns and what our bodies are telling us? Many of our bodies' signals are subtle, and most of us do not take time to slow down and listen to them. Our culture—with its barrage of food, rapid pace, and expectations of immediate fulfillment—doesn't encourage this, and our busy lives don't seem to have any room for it. The sheer amount of stimuli coming at us keeps our attention focused outward, not inward. In our culture, it is just too easy for external cues to override our bodies' signals.

We move through our days paying little heed to what our bodies are telling us—and instead eat in response to external cues. Some people eat by the clock, breaking for lunch every day at 1 P.M. whether or not they're hungry. Some of us are lured as we walk by the break room, home to generous donations from parties past or well-meaning office mates. We pass by the counter that has the jar of chocolates on it (in a clear jar, no doubt!). Or we sit in front of the TV and that commercial comes on advertising the pizza with the impossibly stretchy cheese, and suddenly we're craving pizza, even though we just finished dinner. Research findings note a relationship between being overweight or obese and eating in response to external cues. But there is another option: learning to eat (and stop eating) in response to our *internal* cues.

The heart of mindful eating is tuning in to your body's signals with curiosity and kindness. You might be aware of your patterns with hunger and fullness, or you might have only a fuzzy recognition of them. And even if you are aware of your patterns—*I never eat breakfast, and by the time I eat lunch I feel shaky*—you probably have trouble changing them. That's not unusual. Remember, habits are wired into our brains and bodies over years of practice, but they can be changed with the right tools and supports. One major support system resides within you: your own appetite-regulation system, more commonly known as hunger and fullness signals. Hunger and fullness are multifaceted, with physical, emotional, mental, and cultural factors coming into play. We were born with—and can recultivate—an internal cuing system that is aligned with what our bodies truly need. In this chapter, you'll get better acquainted with your hunger and fullness signals, notice your patterns, and begin to change the habits that aren't serving you well.

Your Mindfulness Toolkit

We're adding new tools to your mindfulness toolkit. In addition to the practices from earlier chapters, in this chapter you'll learn a new exercise to expand your awareness and create the groundwork for healthy choices.

- Hunger-Fullness Scan

Relearning Your Body's Signals

Since we spend most of our time focused externally, it's not surprising that we often miss the quieter cues our bodies use to try to get our attention. One of the principles of integrative medicine is the importance of listening to the innate wisdom of the body. It often speaks to us in whispers. If we're listening, we can respond before mild symptoms turn into serious ones. If we're not listening, our bodies' signals get increasingly loud. This is true for everyday ailments, for stress-related symptoms and conditions, and for the development of chronic illnesses. Our daily experience of hunger and fullness is a microcosm of this phenomenon.

People usually think of hunger and fullness in black and white: you're either hungry or you're not, and you're either full or you're not. In fact, there are gradations of hunger and, even more important, gradations of fullness. There's a spectrum for each. This concept is new to many people—and it's powerful information. Once you know that the gradations exist, you can learn to tune in to them. You did so instinctively as an infant and a young child; relearning those signals and using them as guideposts can help you to change your relationship with food.

Use of the 7-point Hunger-Fullness Scale below, adapted from the work of Linda Craighead, Ph.D., has been shown in clinical research to help people regulate their eating behavior. In our programs, we have found it enormously beneficial in helping people to sense the subtle gradations of hunger and fullness. If you wait too long to start eating or to stop eating, using the scale will support you in creating healthier patterns.

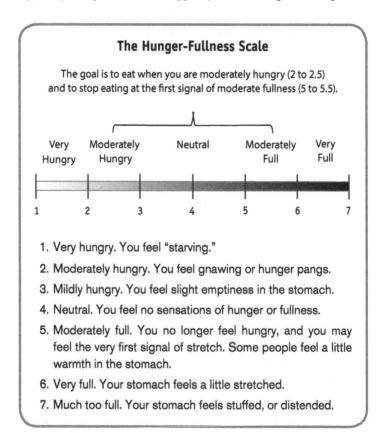

The Hunger-Fullness Scale

The goal is to eat when you are moderately hungry (2 to 2.5) and to stop eating at the first signal of moderate fullness (5 to 5.5).

| Very Hungry | Moderately Hungry | Neutral | Moderately Full | Very Full |

1   2   3   4   5   6   7

1. Very hungry. You feel "starving."
2. Moderately hungry. You feel gnawing or hunger pangs.
3. Mildly hungry. You feel slight emptiness in the stomach.
4. Neutral. You feel no sensations of hunger or fullness.
5. Moderately full. You no longer feel hungry, and you may feel the very first signal of stretch. Some people feel a little warmth in the stomach.
6. Very full. Your stomach feels a little stretched.
7. Much too full. Your stomach feels stuffed, or distended.

On this scale, 1 indicates being extremely hungry, or "starving"—how most people feel after not eating for many waking hours. In this state, you might get a headache and feel weak, light-headed, or jittery; your stomach might actually hurt. And 7 means being extremely full, or stuffed—the classic "Thanksgiving food coma" when you wish you were wearing expandable sweatpants. In this state, your stomach is distended and you feel uncomfortable—potentially sick or nauseous. Note that while extreme hunger and extreme fullness are at opposite ends of the scale, they're both often marked by discomfort (or outright pain), fatigue, and a general feeling of illness.

While we tend to be familiar with the extremes of hunger and fullness, it's getting in touch with the territory in between—moderate hunger and moderate fullness—that can help us change our habits. *What you'll be aiming for is to start eating at 2–2.5 and to stop eating at 5–5.5.* Just like Goldilocks, you want neither too much nor too little. You want to aim for a level of hunger and fullness that's "just right." With moderate hunger, you feel a gnawing or emptiness in the belly, sometimes a pang; your stomach might growl. (Keep in mind that your stomach makes noise during digestion, too, and that noises lower in the gut are likely gas!) When moderately full, many people feel slight warmth in the stomach, the very *first* sensations of its slight stretching, and an absence of pangs or gnawing feelings.

Whereas extreme hunger and fullness are like screams, moderate hunger and fullness are like whispers. The sensations are subtle, and they take practice to notice. Before trying to change anything, practice tuning in to your body's signals with the Hunger-Fullness Scan, below. It's a type of body scan focused specifically on hunger and fullness. The first time you do it, spend about ten minutes—and keep practicing until you get the hang of it. Once you do, you'll start getting a sense of your patterns— still without trying to change them—by doing a quick (ninety-second) Hunger-Fullness Scan before, during, and after meals or anytime you eat.

As with all the exercises in this book, it's critical that you withhold judgment. Think of yourself as a researcher, gathering information and clues about how your body and mind work. You're not trying to *do* anything; you're simply *noticing*. If thoughts or emotions come up, practice the technique we introduced in the last chapter—distinguish the data from the story of the data—this time focused specifically on the sensations of hunger and fullness. The same data can be interpreted in many ways. Take, for example, a mild hunger pang. It's possible to attach numerous stories (thoughts or interpretations) to it. One story might be, *I'd better eat right this second or I'll be famished.* Another: *I can ignore this signal and it will go away.* A third: *I don't need to eat right now, but I should eat within the hour.* Be sure to keep up with your daily mindfulness meditation, which will hone your non-judgment skills.

🔊 Mindfulness Tool: Hunger-Fullness Scan

1. Start by finding the location of your stomach. It is about the size of your fist, and sits right below (not behind) your breastbone and a bit to the left. When you get information from your body right here, it is likely to be a hunger or fullness signal.

2. Get into a comfortable seated position, closing your eyes. At your own pace, start a 20 Breaths practice, just breathing in and out until you feel a sense of looseness and ease.

3. Take a moment to scan your body, noticing any places that may be holding any unnecessary tension, tightness, or stress. Start with your feet, noticing what you feel and allowing any tension to ease. Repeat this process for your legs, then your torso, then your shoulders, then your arms, then your neck, then your jaw and face.

4. Bring your awareness to your stomach or belly. You may want to rest your hand right below your breastbone and over the stomach to help you notice the physical sensations in this part of your body. Notice how your belly rises and falls with each breath. You may notice the texture of your clothes, or the temperature. Just notice whatever is happening.

5. If your mind wanders from the physical sensations of what is happening in this moment, notice what your mind is doing. Is it creating judgments about your body? Old stories or beliefs? Just let them be, and return your attention to the physical experience of your body in this moment.

6. Now direct your awareness into the center of your body. Let your awareness rest gently on the stomach and the sensa-

tions inside. See if you can notice the deeper sensations there. You might notice warmth or coolness, some degree of emptiness or fullness, or movement inside the stomach. Just notice whatever is there—or not there. Remember that there is no right or wrong experience. Simply attend to your stomach with interest and curiosity, wanting to know and observe what your body has to tell you.

7. Notice how hungry or full you are, with 1 being as hungry as possible, 4 being neutral, and 7 being as full as you could possibly be. Remember that these sensations may be very subtle or strong; just make your best estimate of your hunger or fullness rating. Remind yourself that this will take practice over time, so be patient with your best guess for now. No one knows this information better than you.

8. Reflect on the sensations that help you find the rating. And with the next breath, begin to expand your focus back to the room. Then open your eyes.

9. For the next five days, practice the scan as many times as you need to, until you feel you've gotten the hang of it and can do it fairly quickly—in about 90 seconds.

Once you get a handle on this scan, you will begin tracking your hunger and fullness more systematically. First, get used to doing the scan. Later, you will learn to notice your hunger and fullness cues and you'll use those clues to determine where to make shifts that align with your needs. The incredible part is that it will be coming from inside of you. You won't be forcing anything on yourself; rather, you'll be listening deeply to what your body invites you to do.

The Science of Appetite

You might remember from high-school biology class that homeostasis—physiological balance—is the body's natural state.

Our body works to maintain an even keel for basic functions ranging from body temperature to blood pressure. Homeostasis applies to food intake, too: our bodies contain an intricate system designed to regulate our eating, guiding us to eat what is needed to fuel our bodies' energy needs and stop when we've had enough. At the heart of this complex system is an exchange of information between the body and the brain.

An area of the brain called the hypothalamus acts as "command central" for appetite, receiving messages that the body sends out in the form of hormones—some related to hunger and others to fullness. The brain then produces its own hormones that guide us to either eat or stop eating. One of the body's most well-known "hunger hormones" is **ghrelin.** Cells in the stomach and intestines send this hormone to the brain frequently—every thirty minutes. If ghrelin were in charge, we'd eat continuously, but a number of "fullness hormones" have a counterbalancing effect. **Leptin,** produced by fat cells, is one such fullness hormone that has profound effects on food intake over the long term. When things are working properly, leptin's messages override those of ghrelin in the brain, and the result is that we feel full and satisfied until our bodies truly need more food. High levels of leptin may make it easier for people to resist the temptation of high-calorie foods. When we're eating, hormones such as **CCK** (released in response to the presence of protein and fat) increase satiety in the brain—as do stretch receptors in our gut that are triggered when our bellies get distended, about fifteen to twenty minutes into a meal.

Many things can disrupt the body's appetite-regulation system, such as ignoring internal signals and eating too much or too little. Over time, overeating can disrupt the response of both leptin and ghrelin. In addition, when you restrict calories or skip meals, ghrelin's signals happen even more frequently—about every twenty minutes—which can lead to overeating. A third major way we disrupt the body's appetite-regulation system is based on what we eat. Humans evolved to eat whole foods—vegetables and fruit, lean proteins, fats, and whole grains—and we still have the same basic biology. You'll learn more about the health benefits provided by a whole-foods diet in chapter 10, but the important point here is that it supports balance in our appetite-regulation system, while the refined carbohydrates, sugars, and fats found in processed foods that are so abundant in the typical American diet do not. The highly processed sugar known as high-fructose corn syrup, for instance, appears to interfere with body-brain communication—the calories don't register as fullness in the brain.

When people gain excess weight through whichever mechanism, both the brain and individual cells can begin to resist the normal influence of leptin. The upshot of this state, called **leptin resistance,** is that satiety remains elusive even when leptin levels are high. Research indicates that leptin resistance further contributes to obesity and may help to explain why weight loss can be so challenging. Studies suggest, however, that shifting to a whole-foods diet can help "undo" leptin resistance.

Understanding Your Hunger and Fullness Patterns

Once you've learned how to tune in to your body's signals, you can use the Hunger-Fullness Scan to get a sense of your patterns. In the exercise below, you'll spend three days noticing and recording how your body feels before, during, and after every meal or snack, and noting your hunger-fullness rating—*without trying to change anything.* That might sound tedious, but it's only three days—and the information you'll gain is invaluable.

Notice that we are specifically asking you to notice and keep track of *physical* sensations rather than thoughts or emotions. Here's why: Suppose you rate your hunger as 1.5 solely based on feeling extremely irritated (an emotion); while being irritated *may* be a sign of hunger, it could also indicate many other things. Or suppose you rate yourself a 1.5 solely because it's been four hours since you last ate (a thought); without a physical sensation, you really don't know your hunger level. We want you to learn to recognize hunger and fullness from the inside—from the physical sensations that accompany them, which are more consistent and stable indicators than emotions or thoughts. If you are at a hunger-fullness rating of 1.5 because of the intense pangs in your stomach and the headache that's starting (physical sensations), you're on target for identifying the physical sensations we're trying to map.

Tracking Hunger and Fullness (Sample)

Time and place	Food eaten	Before eating	Mid-meal or snack	After eating
		(sensations and H-F rating)		
9:30 A.M., car	Bagel with butter, orange juice	Pangs in stomach (Rating: 2)	Emptiness (Rating: 3)	No longer empty, relief of pangs (Rating: 4.5)
11:30 A.M., break room	M&Ms (big handful)	Slight emptiness (Rating: 3)	No sensation (Rating: 4)	No feelings of emptiness, first sign of stretch at belly (Rating: 5)
1:00 P.M., sub shop near work	Turkey sub and chips, soda	Stomach growling, salivating, feeling of "hole" in stomach (Rating: 1.5)	Warmth in belly, relief of discomfort there (Rating: 5)	Stomach stretched, sleepy (Rating: 6.5)
7 P.M., home	Spaghetti and meatballs, French bread, salad	Pain in stomach, light-headed (Rating: 1)	Warmth, slight stretch in stomach (Rating: 5.5)	Stomach hurts, bloated, low energy (Rating: 7)

Exercise: Track your Hunger and Fullness

1. Copy the column headings in the sample above into your journal or notebook. You'll need to keep it with you for the three days you're doing the exercise. (Create new pages as needed.)

2. Every time you eat, whether it's a meal or a snack, do a quick Hunger-Fullness Scan *before* you eat—without trying to change anything. Record your physical sensations and your hunger-fullness rating in your journal.

3. Do another quick scan *during* the meal or snack—again, without trying to alter your behavior.

4. After the meal or snack, do a final scan, and again, record your physical sensations and your hunger-fullness rating. Also note the time and where you are.

5. Repeat this process for three days, recording your physical sensations and hunger-fullness rating for every meal and snack.

6. After the three days, spend a little time reviewing the data you gathered. What patterns do you notice? Did you tend to wait too long to start eating? Did you tend to wait too long to stop eating (overeat)? Or perhaps you started eating—and kept eating—when you were not hungry at all? Did you notice any new sensations? There's no right or wrong answer. It's the awareness that's important. Record your observations in your journal.

Becoming aware of your patterns with hunger and fullness is an enormous first step. Maintaining this awareness and going deeper—exploring the subtleties of your habits—comes next. We've listed three common patterns below. You might strongly identify with one, or all three might look familiar.

For everyone, **the eventual goal is to eat when you're moderately hungry (2–2.5) and stop when you're moderately full (5–5.5) the vast majority of the time.** How you get there, though, will depend on what your current patterns are.

As you're making changes, remember that charting a different course takes time. Resist the urge to do everything at once; pick one change you can integrate into your life for at least a week before adding a second one. If you identify with multiple patterns, do one tracking exercise at a time rather than trying to track all your patterns at once.

We can't emphasize enough the importance of listening to your body. Your meditation practice will help you recognize when your thoughts or emotions are driving your eating behavior. Your task as a detective is to learn your *body's* signals.

Common Patterns

Pattern 1: Waiting Too Long to *Start* Eating

If you wait until you're extremely hungry to eat—a 1 or 1.5 on the hunger scale—you may find that you tend to wolf down whatever's in sight, regardless of your healthy-eating intentions. Everyone has experienced this at one time or another, but we see it frequently among people in our healthy-eating programs. The culprit here often isn't willpower, but blood sugar.

Extreme hunger leads to a chemical cascade in your body: your blood-sugar level falls, which triggers a stress response in addition to signaling a need to eat NOW. Simply waiting too long to eat can set off an unhealthy spiral of low blood sugar, stress, bad mood, poor decision-making, and overeating or eating whatever is in the immediate vicinity—often something unhealthy from a vending machine, pantry, freezer, or fast-food drive-through. It's not impossible to interrupt this pattern once it's in motion, but it's very difficult. It's kinder to yourself and much healthier to plan ahead—to be prepared with healthier food options and respond to moderate hunger before it's so extreme. Better to understand—and try to avoid—the circumstances that give rise to it.

Many people are unaware of their body's hunger signals until it's "too late," and others hear their body's signals but ignore them. For some people, stopping to eat seems like a waste of time—and hunger an annoyance. Chronic stress is often a culprit in these cases. Others disregard the sensation of hunger because of past events or beliefs they hold. Still others find that they *enjoy* the prolonged experience of hunger, misinterpreting it as a sign of control over the body. (People suffering from anorexia and other restrictive eating disorders often feel this way.)

Whatever the cause, waiting until you're extremely hungry before eating is physiologically stressful to the body. Even if you're eating only once or twice a day, you may unknowingly take in more calories than you burn. Worse still, it's counterproductive. There's evidence that skipping meals is associated with weight gain even if you *don't* consume excess calories over the course of a day. On a biochemical level, your body goes into starvation mode; it receives the message that food is scarce and works to conserve the calories that you do consume, storing more of it as fat for use later. (This is one reason that low-calorie diets don't work.)

Tracker exercise: Instead of waiting until you're at a 1 on the hunger scale, aim to eat when you're at a 2.5. At first, you'll need to do frequent Hunger-Fullness Scans—about every hour—so that you don't miss your body's signals. Pay attention to what 2.5 feels like; get familiar with the physical sensations and write them down. Eventually, you may be able to recognize your body's signals without doing a scan, but you'll need to consciously pay attention to how your body is feeling.

Other changes to explore: If you tend to wait too long to eat, it's vital to keep healthy snacks nearby—think yogurt, nuts, and whole fresh fruit in your office or at home, whole-food granola bars in your car. Get off to a good start each day by eating breakfast, and plan your meals—getting a sense of what time you'll eat and making sure you have healthy food on hand. If you "forget" to eat, or feel like you don't have time, it's also vital to lower your stress levels; you'll learn more about the stress-and-eating cycle in chapter 7.

Insights and Inspirations: Lydia, age 33

I did a lot of sports in high school and college, and back then I really viewed my body as more of a machine than anything else. Food was fuel to keep it running. Now I sit at a desk and I'm lucky if I make it to the gym once a week. I feel really impatient when I get hungry during my workday—I think it's because on some level I think I don't even believe that my body needs food because it doesn't do much. That's irrational, I know. And when I ignore my hunger, I go crazy at night and practically eat the whole kitchen. But I'm learning to pay attention and take my body's needs seriously. I'm finding that keeping my hunger on an even keel keeps my mood on an even keel, too.

Pattern 2: Waiting Too Long to *Stop* Eating

Just as we miss our bodies' hunger signals, we often miss or ignore the signs that we've had enough food. Many of us fall into this pattern— waiting until we're at a 6, 6.5, or 7 on the Hunger-Fullness Scale to stop eating. Often, people with this pattern ignore their bodies' fullness signals and keep eating until the food is gone or the plate is clean.

Several factors can lead to eating past the point of satiety, starting with speed. To get in touch with your body's fullness signals you have to be able to feel those signals, and eating too fast doesn't allow for that. Our brains take about 20 minutes to register the satiety messages coming in from the gut through the hormones leptin, PYY3-36, CCK, and others, which lead to a sensation of fullness. *Twenty minutes.* You can eat a lot of food and consume a lot of calories in twenty minutes. It's easy enough to wolf down a plate of cookies or a foot-long sub in five minutes. That means you don't feel full until you're long past being done—and then you suddenly feel stuffed.

We're designed to eat slowly. But how do you do that when everything in our culture seems to move quickly? In our quest to get more and more done in the same twenty-four hours, we talk, walk, drive, think, type, and *eat* fast. And we often do several of these things simultaneously. Who has time to slow down? And for people prone to emotional eating, eating quickly can be a coping mechanism, an attempt to rapidly produce brain-chemistry changes that mitigate unpleasant feelings (more on that in chapter 7).

The Science of Slowing Down for Weight Loss

Based on what we know about the biology of satiety, it makes sense that the speed at which we eat affects our weight and body-mass index (BMI), and scientists have begun confirming the connection. Researchers at Australia's Department of Human Nutrition spent several years studying the relationship between the pace at which people eat and their BMI. Surveying more than 1,500 middle-aged women about their eating pace, using a five-step scale from "very slowly" to "very quickly," researchers found that the more quickly the women reported eating, the higher their BMI was. Every one-step increase on the scale was associated with a BMI increase of about 2.8 percent, or about 4 pounds of weight gain. Women who reported eating slowly consistently had the lowest BMI.

"Clean-your-plate syndrome" can also lead to overriding satiety signals. As children, many people are told to finish the food on their plate, regardless of how much food is on it and how hungry or full they are. This directive is often a well-intentioned attempt to get active children to eat enough and to avoid wasting food. Sometimes there's a subtext of guilt, as with a parent who implores, "You're not going to eat all the lasagna I made especially for you? I thought it was your favorite." If this sounds familiar to you, your meditation practice will help you cultivate a sense of stable attention to your body and an ability to recognize when a thought—or belief, in this case—is driving your behavior.

It's also helpful to examine the very notion of what it means to be "full." When a container—a cup or a bathtub—is full, it's at capacity;

there's no more room. If you add more water, it starts spilling out. Our stomachs aren't cups or bathtubs; they do stretch to accommodate extra food. But that doesn't mean they're happy about it. Being full or "stuffed" creates a cascade of metabolic effects that can be much more damaging than water on a bathroom floor. These effects are amplified the "fuller" we are—and the more frequently we eat past moderate fullness. Worse, because of the belly-to-brain time lag, our fullness increases after we've stopped eating. Most people think of "full" when there's no more room, but we should stop eating well before that.

Curbing overeating involves shifting your mind-set from "eating until you're full" to eating until you've had just enough. What do we mean by "just enough"? *Just enough* means that you've eaten the right amount to support your body and your brain to function optimally, enough to satisfy your hunger for about four hours. And enough to give you a feeling of satisfaction—and many times, though not always, pleasure. (This concept can be especially confusing and complex for people who overeat. We'll explore it in depth in the next chapter.)

"Enough" is very different from "full"—and generally involves eating significantly less food. Knowing how much food really is enough takes practice and tuning in to your body. (See "Full versus Enough," below.) So, too, does getting comfortable with the whole concept of eating just enough. If you're used to eating until you're full or "stuffed," eating just enough may feel like deprivation at first, even if you know, logically, that the extra food you're accustomed to eating harms you more than helps you. But shifting to *enough* is well worth the effort: **eating quickly and until you're full triples your risk of being overweight.** Our research has shown that for people who overeat, becoming aware of and responding appropriately to their fullness signals are the most important steps in curbing overeating. Be compassionate with yourself as you work on this pattern.

Tracker exercise: While the goal is to stop eating at 5.5 on the fullness scale, this takes practice. Here are three options to help you get there.

1. Halfway through a meal, take two minutes to do the Hunger-Fullness Scan, and note your rating and associated

physical sensations on the tracker. Continue eating until you feel the very first signal of stretch, then stop at a 5.5. Over the next few hours, notice how your body feels. Do this practice for three days and see what you learn. If you find it too difficult to stop at 5.5, then try stopping halfway through your meal to do the Hunger-Fullness Tracker, but wait ten minutes before continuing to eat. See how this helps you stop eating at a 5.5.

2. Eat for five minutes at a slow pace and then stop and wait for fifteen minutes. Do the Hunger-Fullness Scan and rating. If you're still hungry, eat a little more until you're at a 5.5 on the fullness scale.

3. If you are really up for a challenge, try stopping completely at your usual halfway point. What is your fullness rating now? What happens over the next few hours?

Full versus Enough

You know you're full when . . .	You know you've had enough when . . .
Your stomach feels quite stretched.	You feel the very first signal of stretch. Your stomach stops growling.
Your stomach hurts.	You no longer feel hunger pangs or emptiness in your stomach.
You have heartburn.	You feel physically satisfied, possibly a sense of warmth in the stomach.
You feel tired or even sluggish.	You have increased energy.
You feel like you can't move.	You have the energy to take a walk.
You have to unbuckle your pants, and you can't move well.	You're comfortable and are able to move around freely.
It's hard to take a deep breath.	You can easily breathe deeply.

Other changes to explore: Commit to paying attention to your body's fullness signals, and remember that to recognize them, slowing down is paramount. The goal isn't slowness for its own sake, but to allow time to notice, learn, and give your brain and body a chance to register fullness—which in turn gives you information to make choices more easily, leveraging your body's strengths to communicate with you. Spending thirty minutes eating a meal is a minimum to allow your brain to register fullness. That's a dramatic change for most people, though, and is not always realistic given the constraints of our lives. The tracking exercises above offer alternative strategies.

If you're in the "clean plate club," familiarize yourself with healthy portions rather than typical portions (see chapter 11) so that you're able to recognize when your plate is too full. The external visual will help you remember to check inside for the real information. Whenever possible, put less food on your plate—and/or use a smaller plate or bowl. Studies by Cornell University's Brian Wansink, Ph.D., and others have shown that the bigger our plate is, the more we eat. In fact, we eat about 92 percent of what is on our plate, regardless of the plate size. Still, there will probably be times when you're handed a very full plate of food and feel a pressure or expectation to finish it. If you're at a restaurant and are served an enormous portion, ask your server for a to-go container and immediately put half your meal in it. If you're with family or friends and are

---

Insights and Inspirations: Gwen, age 57

I had a really good experience investigating my own hunger and satiety. It made me aware of how often I eat when I'm not actually hungry, and just keep eating past the point of fullness. I now stop and ask myself, "What am I doing here in front of this refrigerator? Am I hungry? And if not, what is going on?" And I end up pushing away a lot of food when I've had enough. It's powerful.

worried about hurting their feelings, it might take practice being asser-
tive about portions.

Reflect on the following questions in your journal: What are the posi-
tives of overeating? And the downsides? How does routinely eating more
than enough undermine you in doing what you want in your life?

Hungry All the Time?

If you feel physically hungry less than 4 hours after your last meal,
what you're eating may need an adjustment. Protein and fat induce
satiety more effectively than carbohydrates do—foods high in protein and fat "stick to your ribs." So if you're eating mainly carbohydrates, you may feel hungry more frequently, particularly if the
carbs are refined. Try incorporating protein and healthy fat during
each meal or snack and see if that makes a difference. As with the
previous pattern, planning is key—keep healthy meals and snacks
on hand.

Pattern 3: Eating Before You're Hungry

Many people who struggle with their weight eat at the slightest sign of
hunger or even when they're not hungry—between 3 and 4 on the scale.
They turn to food well before they're moderately hungry, often *for reasons other than hunger*. It's normal to eat for non-hunger reasons once
in a while, but people who struggle with weight tend to do so regularly.

All the external cues in our culture contribute to this pattern. While
there's plenty of "noise" to distract us from our natural hunger signals,
sometimes they're in overdrive. The fact is, the food industry wants us
to be hungry all the time—or at least to *think* we're hungry. If you're
walking down a city street, or you're on the Internet, or near a TV, or at
the grocery store, you're surrounded by food or images of food. These

triggers cause real physical changes in the body. You may even salivate at these external cues, but that doesn't necessarily mean you are physically hungry. In fact, we recommend that people not use salivation as a sign of physical hunger. (While it's true that you salivate when hungry, you salivate for other reasons, too.) Other external cues include "eating by the clock" (see sidebar below) and being around other people who are eating.

Some of us are prompted to eat when we are not physically hungry by internal triggers. Many of us use food to quell difficult emotions and stress—we'll delve into this important topic in chapter 7. For some, the sensation of hunger, even slight hunger, induces a storm of thoughts and feelings akin to panic. Certain emotions, such as anger and mild to moderate anxiety, have physical manifestations that can mimic hunger.

Whatever the reason, eating when you're not physically hungry confuses your body and can lead to weight gain. Other consequences include feeling out of control with food, disconnected from our bodies, and guilty. Moreover, eating in response to stress or other emotions can be counterproductive for not only your physical health, but your emotional health, too. Instead of coping with stressors in a healthy way, you can remain stuck in a pattern that ultimately makes things worse.

Tracker exercise: Over the next week, when you're mildly hungry—3 or 3.5, even 2.5—in addition to writing your sensations on the tracker, write your thoughts and feelings. See if you can separate the data (what your body sensations are) from your story.

Other changes to explore: Determining whether you're physically hungry takes daily practice. If you tend to eat for emotional reasons, remind yourself that being physically hungry is often distinct from *wanting* to eat; use the Hunger-Fullness Scan to discern the difference. If you realize that you often eat before your body has a chance to get hungry, it's important to explore why you are eating—whether it's due to external cues or internal cues such as thoughts or emotions. Keep your journal with you, and if you're aware that you're eating for a non-hunger reason, note it without judgment.

It also helps to practice getting comfortable with mild and occasionally moderate hunger. That means accepting the fact that sometimes you're going to be hungry, and that's okay—it doesn't mean you have to eat immediately. It might mean that you need to start preparing or arranging for healthy food if you haven't planned ahead, but it doesn't necessarily mean "eat now." Practice your regular Sitting Meditation and separating the data from the story, both of which will help you make healthy choices.

Insights and Inspirations: Sara, age 42

For most of my life, I ate whenever I felt hungry in the slightest. I hated the feeling of hunger. I don't even really know why, except that it felt like a hole that I had to fill, immediately, with whatever food was close at hand. Figuring out which foods would "stick to my ribs" helped, but for me, the most important thing was getting comfortable with the sensation of hunger. I came to understand that it was my body just letting me know what it needed. I didn't have to panic. I started telling myself—literally saying the words in my head or out loud—that I wasn't going to starve, that what I was feeling was "just hunger" and that I would take care of it within the hour. I'd remind myself that the hunger meant my body was working well, letting me know what it needed. And I'd reassure my body that I heard it and that healthy food was on the way. Practicing that has been really liberating.

Eating by the Clock

Sometimes we eat simply because "it's time to eat," regardless of how hungry or full we are. We call this pattern "eating by the clock," and there's a lot in our family, work schedules, and the larger culture that encourages it.

If you see this pattern in yourself, be sure to check in with your hunger and fullness signals at mealtimes. When work schedules prevent you from being able to respond to physical hunger cues easily, more planning is required. You have to work backward to figure out what healthy sources of carbohydrates, fat, and protein will get you through the time period when you can't respond well to hunger. (You'll learn more about this in chapter 10.) For example, if your lunch break is at noon and you don't eat dinner until 7:30, consider what protein, healthy fats, and whole fruits and vegetables for lunch will give you enough fuel to get you through the seven-hour period between lunch and dinner. You are likely to need a quick snack, so having almonds or a low-fat cheese stick readily available is key.

It's easier to align eating with your physical hunger and fullness in personal time, but consider social eating. Can you imagine telling family or friends that you'll join them at the table to visit but aren't going to eat until you are hungry? Can you imagine attending social engagements without eating, or eating just a little, if you're not hungry? This might feel awkward at first, but it's an important part of self-care and key to breaking the "eating by the clock" pattern.

Insights and Inspirations: Craig, age 54

I've been eating breakfast at 7:30, lunch at noon, and dinner at 6:00 P.M. for as long as I can remember. That's what we did growing up, and that's what I do now. It honestly never occurred to me to "eat when I'm hungry" or to not eat at mealtime if I wasn't hungry. When I'd feel hungry between meals, I'd just tell myself it wasn't time to eat and wait it out. But when I started paying attention, I realized that I was actually pretty uncomfortable a lot of the time.

Hunger and Emotions

In the West, we tend to ascribe emotions to the purview of the mind—and to treat them as being totally distinct from the body. The idea that the mind and body are separate, known as mind-body dualism, originated with 17th-century philosopher René Descartes, who famously pronounced, "I think, therefore I am." Modern Western medicine was built on this duality, with an exclusive focus on the body's chemistry and skepticism about the links between our emotions and our physical health.

In fact, the mind and body are inextricably linked—and emotions are as much a physical experience as a mental one. Learning to discern the physiological indication of an emotion from the body's indication that it is hungry will become a key part of responding well to your hunger and fullness cues. Anger, for instance, can cause a burning sensation in the abdomen, and fear can cause a fluttering in the belly. And everyone is different; one person might experience fear in her lower belly, while another feels it in her chest. So if you don't tune in to your own signals of how you're really feeling emotionally, you might assume you're hungry and act accordingly when you're actually experiencing an emotion that does not indicate the need to eat.

Separating out emotions from physical signals that indicate hunger, fullness, or other physical needs (e.g., fatigue, indicating a need for rest) is perhaps the most challenging part of learning to use your body's wisdom. Hence, we've devoted a whole chapter to it, chapter 7. We'll turn there after you've gotten more practice discerning your physical signals for hunger and fullness.

Staying the Course

Awareness of your hunger and fullness patterns is one of the foundations of mindful eating. The information you've gathered is empowering. You might have learned, for instance, that you consistently override your fullness signals. You might have realized that you're so stressed out that you don't prioritize meal planning and end up getting so hungry that you lose control. Keep listening. The more practice you have paying attention to your body's signals, the easier it will be to listen and distinguish your real needs: do you need food or rest? Food or a stress break? Food or company? Food or something interesting and meaningful to do?

You've been tracking when you start eating, and when you stop, in your journal. Use the Hunger-Fullness Scan before each time you eat, and as you collect data on yourself, remember your intention. Once you see your patterns, decide what small shift to make next. For example, if you typically skip breakfast, try eating a regular small and healthy one—a piece of whole-grain toast with almond butter, for instance. If you typically eat until a 6.5, try stopping at 6 for a week. Support whatever changes you decide to make by creating a set of goals for sustainable change and tracking your behavior.

Here's what's universal: if you want to use the incredible innate system your body already has to change your eating patterns, you have to start paying attention to your body and prioritizing its well-being. **Keep in mind that your ability to enjoy a meal is not related to how much you eat.** Keep your values and goals at the forefront of your mind and remember that you're honoring your body by listening to it.

CHAPTER 6

The Pleasure Principle

"The banquet is in the first bite."

—Michael Pollan

ood is powerfully connected to our sensory experiences and therefore to our memories. We remember the way it looks, how we felt eating it, the way it tastes. From sweet to salty, creamy to crunchy, the flavors and textures of food linger on the tongue and transport the mouth and the mind to a happy place. It may be the creamy sweetness of ice cream that moves you—or the bittersweet richness of chocolate, the simple tart pop of fresh berries, or the crispy, chewy goodness of roast chicken. Or all of the above, and more. Food tastes *good*. It's supposed to.

Along with hunger, the enjoyment of flavor is one of our basic motivations for eating—a "driver," in health-psychology terms. And yet, the appreciation of flavor is a double-edged sword. Some people who struggle with eating habits and weight see their taste buds as their downfall. "If I could just forget about the taste of onion rings, I think everything else would fall into place," Lydia, age 30, said during one of our programs, prompting laughter from the rest of the room. "I'm not kidding!"

It might seem counterintuitive, but learning to tune in to the flavor of food can help to curb overeating and guide you toward healthier choices. Mindless eating habits—eating very quickly or while watching TV, driving, or multitasking, for example—short-circuit not only our hunger and fullness signals, as you learned in the last chapter, but also our experience of flavor. So if you wolf down a Snickers bar on the way home from the grocery store, or eat a bowl of pasta and sauce in front of the TV, you hardly taste what you're eating. When that happens, *your brain still seeks satisfaction.* So what do you do? Eat more. What's missing is a full experience of eating, informed by your senses. **The missing ingredient is attention, not more food.** We miss the experience when we pay attention to other things simultaneously. The solution? Mindful awareness of every aspect of the food itself. By learning to deepen your experience of taste, you can get flavor to work in your favor. This gives you one more tool in your mindfulness toolkit.

What the Science Says: The Power of Your Beliefs

Our beliefs about food affect not only the choices we make, but also our *biology.* Researchers at Yale University gave study participants two shakes: one was labeled a high-fat, 620-calorie "indulgent" shake, the other a low-fat, 130-calorie "sensi-shake." In fact, the two shakes were identical. Yet the participants' belief that one was an indulgence—"heaven in a bottle," the label noted—while the other was a healthier choice had powerful effects on their bodies' response to the shakes. Levels of ghrelin, a hormone that stimulates appetite, rose steeply in anticipation of drinking the "indulgent" shake and then fell sharply afterward, indicating that the drink was satisfying. With the "sensible" shake, ghrelin levels stayed relatively flat or rose only slightly in anticipation, and they did not fall steeply afterward, indicating that the drink was not satisfying. The shake contents were the same, but participants' beliefs changed their appetite-regulation hormones.

Wired for Flavor

Satiety—the satisfied feeling of having had enough food—triggers us to stop eating. In the last chapter we talked about one type of satiety, fullness. You learned that one of the ways that we know we have had enough food is through physical sensation—the way our bodies, especially our stomachs, feel while we're eating or afterward—and you practiced slowing down and tuning in to those sensations. Another type of satiety is called "taste satiety," a term used by Jean Kristeller to make the concept of sensory-specific satiety easier to understand. Taste satiety is not about the stomach, but about the tongue.

When we eat food with a particular flavor—sweet, salty, sour, or bitter—the pleasure we receive from it builds, peaks, and then starts to decline. That peak prior to the decline is taste satiety—the sensation that we've had enough of a particular flavor. You know the sensation: that fourth bite of cheesecake when it goes from heavenly to neutral. When that shift happens, the neural activity in the brain shifts. Studies show that taste satiety affects brain activity in our hypothalamus, which controls our appetite, and our prefrontal cortex, which controls most aspects of our behavior. A number of factors influence taste satiety, including the size of the bites we take, how physically hungry we are, the speed at which we eat, whether we're eating whole or processed food, and the flavor mix in each food. When it's working normally, our taste satiety mechanisms tell us we've "had enough" of a particular flavor, but you have to slow down and pay attention to get the message.

Taste satiety is designed to encourage interest in eating a variety of foods for nutritional balance. If you're hungry when you start eating, you'll generally reach taste satiety well before you feel fullness signals; if you're eating a balanced, healthy meal, taste satiety can help you to eat some of everything on your plate. (It's trickier when you're eating processed foods specifically designed to override taste satiety, as we'll explain below.) Understanding how taste satiety works is also a key to "pleasure eating"—those times when you want something sweet after dinner or you're craving the salty, creamy flavor of your favorite cheese.

Your Mindfulness Toolkit

We're adding new tools into your mindfulness toolkit. In addition to the practices from earlier chapters, in this chapter you'll learn another exercise to expand your awareness and lay the groundwork for getting more pleasure from less food.

• Taste Awareness

🔊 Mindfulness Tool: Taste Awareness (Single Food)

When you slow down and focus on flavor, your experience of eating can change radically. This exercise will help you become more aware of different tastes and give you a better sense of when you have eaten enough of a specific food. For example, a very small amount of a highly sweetened food may be enough to reach taste satiety.

For this exercise, you'll need a single chocolate kiss. Do this exercise when you are not hungry so you can fully focus on flavor. It takes about twenty minutes and should be done alone in a quiet place.

1. Begin by placing a single chocolate kiss in front of you, out of your hands. Allow your eyes to close, or find a downward gaze if closing your eyes feels too uncomfortable. Rest your hands on your stomach, inviting four or five deep, easy breaths.

2. Allow your body to rest while you move your attention to your stomach and mouth. Notice any physical sensations you have at this time. Notice any thoughts you have. Notice any emotions. Be aware of the difference between physical sensations on the one hand and thoughts or emotions on the other. Whatever you experience, just observe it, trying not to judge or criticize it. Just notice whatever you are experiencing. Don't try to change it; just notice, trying to separate out the emotion or thought from physical sensa-

tions. If you don't sense any particular sensations, feelings, or thoughts, that's okay too.

3. Now, in the next breath, or the one after that, allow your eyes to fully open. Take the piece of chocolate in your hand and unwrap it gently. Continue to be aware of any thoughts or emotions that pass through your mind. Look at the chocolate, holding it in your open palm, noticing it as if this were the first time you had ever seen chocolate. If you were a painter, how would you paint it? Notice the shape, the size, the colors, the way the light reflects on it.

4. Now move your attention to the smell of the chocolate. Place it under your nose, close your eyes again, and just notice the scent. Where in your nose do you smell the chocolate? What aspects of it can you smell? Milk? Vanilla? Tobacco or an earthy scent? Notice all you can about the scent.

5. Now rub the kiss on your lips so you get just a hint of flavor. Allow your eyes to remain closed. What do you taste? What do you notice about the texture? Is it smooth or gritty? Melting or not? Be aware of all the intricacies in this one chocolate kiss.

6. Now place the chocolate on your tongue, but do not bite it. What do you now notice about the flavor? Move it around your mouth. Does it taste different in different parts of your mouth? Allow it to melt on your tongue. What do you notice as it melts? Just allow yourself to be fully present. What do you notice about your saliva? About your mouth itself? Does the flavor change over time, as it melts? In what way?

7. Take as long as you like to allow the chocolate to melt and to fully experience the sensations of biting and eating it. Can you feel it move out of your mouth, into your throat? Into your stomach? Be aware of any thoughts or emotions that pass through, distinguishing them from a sensation like taste.

When you have fully finished the chocolate kiss, allow your eyes to open and take a few moments to note any observations of the experience. What if you ate like this most of the time?

The Physics of Flavor

Clients are often surprised at how quickly they reach taste satisfaction when they slow down and really pay attention to flavor. Most reach taste satiety with a single kiss, and after that, the flavor diminishes. Knowing that you can get as much satisfaction from one piece of chocolate as from ten is powerful information, especially when dealing with cravings.

Like many people, Bonnie, age 34, craved chocolate frequently, especially when she was tired or stressed. "I used to eat a whole candy bar—fast. And then sometimes another one," she said. "It was like I couldn't get enough." In one of our programs, she applied the taste satiety exercise to a piece of chocolate and found it transformative. "When I slowed down and really focused, I was able to enjoy three bites of chocolate more than my usual candy-bar binge. And no stomachache. And no guilt!" Instead of buying candy bars, she bought individually wrapped squares of her favorite dark chocolate. She still loves chocolate, but now, when she experiences a craving, she eats a single square slowly and with attention. "It doesn't feel like denying myself," she says. "It actually feels like *more* of an indulgence."

Could taking a couple of bites with full attention truly help you? Scientists have been studying taste satiety for decades, so there's a solid body of research on variables and techniques that influence how satisfied you are by a given meal or snack. Even though everyday eating is rarely as attentive as it was in the exercise above, you can use taste satiety as a tool for healthy eating by keeping the following things in mind:

Speed. The speed at which you eat can affect how satisfied you'll be. In one study that compared people's experience of eating ice cream slowly (taking thirty minutes) versus quickly (in five minutes), eating slowly led to significantly higher levels of a satiety hormone called peptide YY, or PYY, for several hours after the ice cream was eaten. This suggests that eating slowly keeps you satisfied longer—which can help to reduce your overall food intake. In our own clinical research and practice, we've seen that to notice taste changes, you have to slow the eating process way down, and focus deeply.

How to apply it: Be intentional about slowing down. For "pleasure food" that you tend to eat quickly, start by doing the Taste Awareness exercise with the food. As you continue eating, put down your fork (or the food, if it's a finger food) between bites and ask yourself if you've had enough.

Bite size. A cookie has the same number of calories whether you eat it in three bites or in ten. But how satisfied you'll feel from that cookie—and how much you end up eating—can vary radically, depending not just on the speed of your eating but also on the size of your bites. What's the explanation? Research suggests that satiety is reached sooner and *less total food is eaten* when smaller bites are taken. Even though the caloric contents are the same, you get more sensory pleasure from more bites, so you reach taste satiety sooner.

How to apply it: It's easy to put this principle into practice. When you're eating an afternoon snack or a post-dinner dessert, try breaking or cutting your food into smaller bites and attending to the flavor of each bite. As with the slowing-down advice above, after each bite, ask yourself if you've had enough—and when you have, stop. Wait fifteen to twenty minutes to decide whether you really want more.

Simple versus complex flavors. Research and our clinical experience show that people reach taste satiety more quickly with one flavor than with multiple flavors. One landmark study showed that when people were given "pure sweet," such as sugar water, they reached their taste satiety peak on the third or fourth sip—much more quickly than you might think. Some people do *not* seem to reach taste satiety after several bites of a "pure" flavor like sweet or salty, however, as described in "Taste Satiety and Weight Gain," below.

When complex flavors are involved, as they often are, it takes longer to reach taste satiety. Consider the salty-sweet mix of a Thai stir-fry, the contrast of peanut butter and chocolate that Reese's made famous, or the salted caramel trend in desserts. As the flavors play in your mouth, your taste buds might start to reach sweet satiety but then get hit with salt, then back to sweet, and so on. It's the difference between listening to a piece of music in its entirety (satisfying) and listening to three overlapping songs (confusing). The contrast is lovely but also delays taste satiety.

What the Science Says: Taste Satiety and Weight Gain

Some studies suggest that obesity may affect taste satiety, diminishing sensitivity to both sweet and fatty flavors. One recent study showed that obese children have less sensitive taste buds than normal-weight children. The causality behind these associations isn't known, but given that the same foods that can lead to weight gain—sweet or fatty convenience foods—can also reduce taste sensitivity, the link between obesity and reduced taste satiety makes sense. We've found, though, that people all along the weight spectrum can shift their experience of taste satiety by paying attention to flavor. Moreover, research shows that losing weight incrementally shifts the experience of satiety. So if you are trying to lose weight, continue to practice the taste satiety exercises to check in with your body and your brain, and note the results in your journal. Pay attention to how your experience of certain foods changes over time.

How to apply it. It's likely that many of your favorite meals have more than one flavor note. With practice, you can get a handle on complex-flavor satiety. But for now, as much as possible, aim for simpler meals in which you're able to separate out flavors, and eat one food at a time. Instead of eating sweet-and-sour chicken, for instance, eat baked chicken with miso soup and a sweet potato—and eat each item separately so that you can tune in to the flavor. When you do eat complex-flavor foods, especially those that are high in caloric density or meant as occasional treats, try slowing way down and noticing shifts in the flavors during each bite (e.g., notice more sweet, less salt, or the opposite). You will notice your satiety more quickly. As you'll see below, avoiding processed food goes a long way toward simplifying your flavor palate.

Whole versus processed. Research shows that compared with whole foods, foods that are heavily processed take a long time to register in terms of taste satiety. In other words, when you're eating flavored tortilla chips, frozen pizza with many toppings, or a candy bar, it takes a long time to feel satisfied even if you're eating slowly. This is no accident.

Food companies are well versed in the science of taste satiety and use it to their advantage, manipulating flavor and texture both to compensate for processing techniques that diminish flavor, such as dehydrating and freezing, and to create what's known as "hyperpalatability." Processed foods—snacks, desserts, meals, condiments, and beverages—are often engineered to have complex flavor combinations that create an almost never-ending satiety loop. And as you learned earlier, when you're not satisfied, you keep eating.

Processed foods undermine our satiety experience in other ways, too. Food companies have taken the flavors sweet and salty to a whole new level, dosing packaged goods with immense amounts of refined sweeteners and salt. When you eat extreme levels of sweet and salty food regularly, that's what you expect when you eat, and your taste buds lose their sensitivity and require increasing levels of flavor to achieve the same level of satisfaction.

There's evidence that on a chemical level, some of the sweeteners used in packaged foods, both calorie-laden varieties and low- or no-calorie sweeteners, don't register in our satiety center in the way that natural sugars do. Whereas glucose (natural sugar) is transported to the brain and provides satiety signals, high-fructose corn syrup, though caloric, does not enter brain tissues and therefore does not signal satiety. In one recent study, when people were given the no-calorie artificial sweetener sucralose, levels of PYY and other satiety-related peptides did not change.

Processed foods are loaded with sodium and artificial flavors not only to create a compelling flavor, but also to mask the bitter or bland flavors of chemical preservatives and other artificial ingredients. In our mindful-eating classes, participants do an exercise in which they lick the flavor coating off a Dorito. They generally report that the chip underneath has no flavor.

However, processed foods need not ruin your experience of flavor forever. You can recalibrate your taste satiety back to a normal, healthy experience of sweet and salty by shifting toward a whole-foods diet, which provides more satiety per calorie than highly refined and processed foods. Since whole foods typically require more chewing than processed foods do, they tend to spend more time in your mouth. This increased "oral-sensory stimulation" may lead to an increased release of gut satiety hormones.

Depending on how long you've been eating processed food and how much of it you consume, recalibrating your taste satiety may take effort and patience. In working with hundreds of clients over the years, we've found that it takes at least two weeks to get comfortable eating a diet that does not include refined sugar (and longer for a diet lower in fat). When you do, however, the natural sweetness of foods such as fruit gets much more intense.

How to apply it: Make a list of the processed and fast foods that you consume on a regular basis. Are there any whose flavors you crave? Think about whether you are willing to give that up for two weeks. What healthy alternative can you substitute? See the chart below for ideas.

Flavors to Savor

	Instead of . . .	Try . . .
Sweet	Cookies and other baked goods, candy bars, ice cream	Berries, grapes, bananas, square of dark chocolate
Salty	Potato chips	Miso soup, celery and organic peanut butter (with salt but no added sugar)
Sour	Sour candy, packaged lemonade	Fresh-squeezed lemonade
Umami	Soups and frozen meals containing MSG	Stir-fry with shiitake mushrooms and garlic, piece of cheese

Insights and Inspirations: Sam, age 36

As a teenager I got addicted to barbecue potato chips, and even as an adult, I kept a stash of them in my desk drawer at work and could easily power through half a bag, especially in the middle of the afternoon. Doing a mindful-eating exercise with them was radical. Once I licked off the fake flavoring, the chip underneath tasted awful, like cardboard. They lost their appeal after that. Now when I see them, "flavored cardboard" pops into my head.

Solid versus liquid. Some 18 percent of our calories come from liquids, many of them high-calorie sodas, juices, sports drinks, and other processed beverages. These "liquid calories" are a huge culprit in the obesity epidemic and a prime target for anyone trying to manage weight. In fact, a recent Johns Hopkins study showed that reducing calories from beverages leads to greater weight loss than reducing calories from food. Here's what to keep in mind: while beverages may quench your thirst, *they aren't very effective at satisfying either hunger or taste satiety.* When you consume liquids, normal taste-satiety mechanisms don't kick in the way they do with solid food. Remember the link between oral-sensory stimulation and satiety described earlier? Compared with solid foods of the same calorie amount, liquids provide less oral-sensory stimulation and therefore don't provoke the "I've had enough of that flavor" sensation that prompts us to stop. This makes sense—liquids don't spend as much time in your mouth (i.e., on your taste buds) as food does. Sugary drinks are also a huge factor in ratcheting up our expectations of sweetness. As for fullness, beverages have much less fiber and therefore move through our digestive system more quickly, prompting rapid changes in blood sugar. They essentially bypass multiple aspects of the body's appetite-regulation system.

If you think you can have the best of both worlds by drinking low- or no-calorie drinks with artificial sweeteners, think again. Remember, artificial sweeteners don't register satiety (and drinking diet soft drinks may contribute to weight gain and a host of health woes). When you're incorporating satiety awareness, keep in mind that sweet drinks—caloric or not—confuse your brain and your body, and the healthiest beverage is the most basic: water.

Insights and Inspirations: Susan, age 58

When I tuned in to taste, I started tasting things more intensely than usual. In terms of flavor, I realized I liked some things that I hardly ever eat, like salad. And some of the things I eat all the time, I don't like at all. Like meat—I don't really like it all that much.

In the Taste Awareness exercise below, you'll practice eating mindfully, with your attention tuned in to flavor. This time, you'll notice contrasts in flavor as well as your personal preferences.

Mindfulness Tool: Taste Awareness (Multiple Foods)

For this exercise you'll need two grapes cut in half and two–three potato chips. Set these on a small plate and put the rest away before beginning. Again, it's important to do this exercise when you are *not hungry* so you'll be able to focus exclusively on flavor rather than also feeling the drive from physical hunger. Do the exercise in a quiet room, and give yourself about twenty minutes.

1. Do a Mini-Meditation (page 78) or 20 Breaths (page 69) to get present.

2. Lift a grape half a few inches from your nose and smell it. Notice the scent and your response.

3. Next, place the grape half in your mouth and close your eyes. Before you bite into it, spend a couple of minutes roll-

ing it around in your mouth. Notice the different textures and flavors. Notice whether or not your mouth starts to salivate.

4. Slowly bite into the grape just once. What flavors do you notice? Where in your mouth do you taste it? How does the texture change?

5. Then slowly begin to chew the grape (but do not swallow). Notice how the flavor and texture change in your mouth. Between chews, allow the remaining food to rest on your tongue and notice the flavor changes.

6. On the basis of flavor, ask yourself whether you've had enough or you want another piece of grape. Does your mouth feel "quenched"? Is the flavor still appealing? If you want more, pick up the other grape half and repeat steps 2 through 6.

7. Allow yourself to swallow and clear your mouth completely; expand your awareness to your entire body. What else has shifted?

8. Now pick up a single potato chip and smell it. Close your eyes and notice all you can about the scent.

9. Gently suck the edges without biting the chip. Notice the salt and/or other spices. Just let those sit on your tongue while you feel their intensity.

10. When you're ready, take a single bite of the chip and move it around your mouth, being careful not to bite it further yet. Allowing all the salts and fats to fill your mouth, what do you notice about the texture of the chip and the flavor as it stays in your mouth? After you've noticed changes in the texture, feel free to swallow it.

11. Next, take a second bite and very slowly chew, observing all changes in flavor and texture. Decide if you want a third bite, and if so, continue in this manner—very slowly, fully noticing.

Spend a few minutes writing in your journal about your experience. At what point did you experience satiety with the grape? The chip? Was it sooner or later than you expected? Think about how you decided when to stop eating the grape halves and the chips.

Be a Connoisseur

Whether you consider yourself a healthy eater or a "junk-food junkie," and whatever flavors or particular foods are your weakness, you can learn a lot from adopting a connoisseur's approach. Whether you're eating a salad or a Snickers bar, practice shifting the way that you attend to flavor. This means slowing down and tuning in to the first few bites of whatever you're eating. You can do this whether you're alone in a quiet room or with a big group in a noisy restaurant.

Using taste satiety is very helpful for cravings. If you're craving a cookie, for instance, you can certainly try to wait out the craving or substitute something naturally sweet. But you can also go ahead and have the cookie, eating it slowly and in small bites, with great attention and mindfulness. Focus your senses on its mouthfeel, texture, and flavor—and ask yourself after each bite whether you've had enough. You'll likely get just as much satisfaction from a few bites as from the whole thing—and you'll miss out on the negative consequences of overeating.

Lydia, who had a weakness for onion rings, practiced eating them mindfully instead, attending to flavor. Two things happened. "I found that I could eat two onion rings really mindfully and get a lot of satisfaction out of them," she said. And by slowing way down, instead of gobbling them quickly, she got to experience what *cold* onion rings tasted like: soggy and unappealing. "It was kind of heartbreaking," she said. But by experiencing her former obsession as unpleasant, she found that she stopped obsessing about onion rings.

Taste satiety is useful during healthy meals and snacks, too, as a tool to help curb overeating and encourage nutritional balance. Suppose you are eating a meal of curried lentils, sautéed spinach and cauliflower, and roasted tomatoes. Along with using your skills discerning hunger and fullness, tune in to the flavors on your plate. Stop eating the food that you feel satiated with, and eat what you are still hungry for. Stop eating the lentils but have more spinach, or stop the tomatoes but have more lentils.

Adopt a sense of curiosity as you experiment with taste satiety. You may come to appreciate vegetables you never had a liking for and taste some off-putting flavors that you never noticed in processed foods or fast food. Our bodies, including our taste buds, get used to what they get, and they adapt. But this takes time. And the process is not only about the revelation of processed-food flavors, but includes whole-food flavors, too. In attending to taste, you might realize that you really *don't* like plain brown rice, but that with the right spices or cooking techniques, you do. As with other aspects of mindfulness, increasing your awareness of flavor opens up new possibilities and helps to enrich the process of making choices.

CHAPTER 7

A Cure for Emotional Eating

"Stress cannot exist in the presence of a pie."

—David Mamet

As you now know, our immediate environments, constant advertising, and our food histories all influence our daily habits—and eventually our weight and our health. But some of the most powerful culprits are invisible. For a lot of people, undercurrents of stress and negative feelings—which often lie outside of conscious awareness—play a large part in determining what, when, and how much we eat.

We've all been there: You hang up from a difficult phone call with anger coursing through you or sadness weighing you down, and before you know it, you've downed not one but *three* brownies. Or you're trying to meet a deadline at work and find yourself munching through an entire bag of Cheetos. On the flip side, when sadness or anxiety hits us really hard—from a heartbreaking loss, an awful argument with someone we love, or pre-presentation jitters, for instance—we often feel unable to eat.

As an isolated incident, eating (or not eating) in response to stress or difficult emotions is natural. Everyone does it occasionally, and as clinicians we consider it a part of normal eating behavior, not something that interferes with life or harms our health. The problem comes when eating becomes the *primary* source of comfort, coping, or pleasure.

Why is eating such a common response to stress? Part of it is chemistry, but on the most obvious level, food provides immediate gratification, distracts us from negative thoughts or emotions, doesn't "talk back," and is always there. The downside is that the benefits are usually brief, while the negative effects are longer lasting in terms of weight and health. Chronic comfort eating is often followed by a backlash of guilt or shame, which, as we've emphasized, counteracts healthy change. And when you engage in comfort eating repeatedly, it reinforces a pattern of eating for non-hunger reasons. On top of all that, when you reflexively turn to food to feel better, you aren't doing anything to solve the issue at hand, whether that's a strained relationship or financial trouble. As we say frequently in our programs, *food is very good at comforting you in the moment—but not so good at solving your problems.* We've had some clients tape that truism on their refrigerator or pantry door as a reminder.

For a lot of people, emotional and stress-related eating is a packaged response that seems to "just happen" before they have a choice, almost like a reflex. "When I'm stressed, I reach for potato chips the way my husband reaches for a cigarette," said Megan, age 39, in one of our classes. This comparison makes sense, both in terms of the way comfort eating gets encoded into neural pathways and in terms of the drug-like biochemical changes that certain foods can prompt. Both consciously and unconsciously, people use food to regulate their moods and manage stress.

These patterns lie at the heart of unhealthy eating habits for a lot of people—and it's the aspect of weight loss that most conventional diet plans fail to acknowledge. But mindfulness provides a way through stress-related eating. As with all automatic behavior, changing patterns starts with awareness, using the skills you've learned to slow down and notice what is really going on in your body and in your mind. As you'll find out, it's possible to take apart your reactions and examine the underlying emotions, thoughts, and physical sensations that, bundled together, prompt you to eat. Once you've "unbundled" a reaction, it loses some of its power, and new, healthier ways to cope emerge. The process we'll guide you through in this chapter is ultimately a call to look at, and care for, your whole self.

Insights and Inspirations: Nora, age 43

Every night is the same: after the dishes are done and my kids are in bed, the coffee ice cream comes out and I sit in front of the TV with a large bowl of it and my favorite spoon. It's my first chance to relax all day; it's my reward. And unlike the rest of my day, the rest of my life, it's such a pure pleasure experience—so sweet and creamy. It's not complicated, and it's never disappointing. Sometimes I think, "This is love." Honestly, it really is like the Platonic ideal of love, just pure goodness and pleasure. Of course I know that this nightly ritual probably has something to do with the number on the scale getting bigger—and my pants getting tighter. But at night on my couch with my ice cream, everything is okay, everything is good.

A Mindful Approach to Emotions

In chapter 4, you learned that mindfulness teaches a middle road to working with emotions, between the extremes of suppressing them and getting overwhelmed by them. Both of these extremes can lead to unhealthy eating behaviors. But as with thoughts, when we practice meditation regularly, we're able to experience emotions while maintaining a valuable distance. That distance allows for a different perspective and a different response.

Happiness and laughter are generally more enjoyable than tears and anger. But *all* primary emotions—anger, sadness, joy, fear, and surprise—evolved for specific reasons and serve an important purpose in our lives. Fear and anger, for example, are designed to protect us from danger by mobilizing our fight-or-flight response. When we experience loss, allowing ourselves to feel sadness can prompt us to reach out to someone for comfort—an "affiliation response," in psychologist-speak, which is an important part of the healing process. On a day-to-day level, negative emotions can function as our internal warning system, a sign that something is out of balance in our world and that we may need to take action. Stuffing down your underlying emotions with food is like turning off a fire alarm when a fire is burning.

That doesn't mean that every time you experience a powerful emotion, you need to do something in the moment. When you're on the "middle road," you're able to decide how to respond to emotions *wisely*, rather than *reactively*, by using your internal resources to consider factors that the automatic emotional response doesn't allow for. Rather than suppressing or distracting us from negative emotions, mindfulness teaches us to welcome them and be curious: *Okay, I feel anger—why? What could that mean? Will it subside if I don't agitate it? Does it signal that there is something I need to change? Is that something external to me, such as the situation I'm in? Or is it about the way I perceive things or react?*

Another important question to ask is, "What is my true need in this situation?" The concept of **true needs** is based on the fact that our deeper, underlying need is often at odds with what we want in the moment—our **immediate need.** Our immediate needs, driven by the brain's powerful limbic system, are often to seek comfort, pleasure, or instant release from difficult emotions; their voice is usually some variation of "I want what I want, now!" Your true needs, on the other hand, are aligned with your long-term goals and values. In chapter 9, we'll go into more depth about how to identify and act on true needs. But simply asking the questions "What is my true need right now?" and "What steps can I take to address that true need?"—and listening for the answers—can have powerful effects.

Take Kylie, age 33, who felt perpetually resentful at work because she worked long hours and produced good work but hadn't had a raise in more than three years. Part of her coping response was eating a bag of peanut M&Ms every night while scrolling through online shopping sites. Through mindfulness, she realized that the underlying emotion—anger—was trying to get her attention so that she would make a change.

She also realized that by chronically using food to cope with her feelings, she was responding to an immediate need for comfort but that eating candy was not going to solve the problem. She got in touch with her core values, two of which were diligence and fairness, and realized that being underpaid for her hard work seemed deeply unfair—and that that sense was not likely to go away if she stayed in her current situation. Even though she couldn't control the outcome, she could take action to respond to her true need. Kylie scheduled a meeting with her boss to discuss her performance and ask for a raise.

Identifying Your Emotions

Some people know exactly how they're feeling emotionally (even if they don't always respond to their emotions in healthy ways). But many people don't, for the simple reason that they were never taught to identify or distinguish between their emotions by their families or their cultures. As mentioned earlier, negative emotions are often discounted or discouraged. As we described in chapter 5, different emotions manifest in the body in different ways, and getting in touch with these physical sensations can help you learn to recognize your feelings. And since emotions can be complicated and layered, even those who *are* in touch with their feelings can benefit from the mapping exercise that follows. You may tap into some difficult emotions while doing this exercise, so carve out some private space and sufficient time (about a half hour) for it.

🔊 Exercise: Mapping Your Emotions

People manifest emotions in different ways. One person might experience fear as a racing heart, another as a cold feeling in the pit of her stomach, and another as a tense feeling in her throat. When doing this exercise, release expectations of what you "should" feel; instead, listen to your body.

1. Sit comfortably with your eyes closed and spend a few minutes meditating.

2. Think of an incident in your life that made you angry. Don't choose a hugely upsetting event to practice with; instead, recall an event or situation that made you fairly angry but not furious. Be very specific, recalling as many details as possible about the incident. It may help to mentally transport yourself back to that incident until, as much as possible, you feel like you are reexperiencing the emotion. Do you notice any physical reactions? If not, scan your body with curiosity—how does your chest feel? Your upper abdomen? Your lower abdomen? Your shoulders? Your jaw? Your forehead? Once you've identified where in the body you experience anger, open your eyes and jot down a few notes about it.

3. Again, sit comfortably with your eyes closed and spend a few minutes meditating. It's important to resettle yourself before moving on in this exercise. At a minimum, do a 20 Breaths meditation. When you're ready, remember a specific incident when you were sad—after the loss of a relationship, or a falling-out with a friend. Again, don't choose the most devastating loss to practice with. As before, be as specific as possible. Do a scan and notice how your body responds. Where do you feel the emotion in your body? How does your chest feel? Your abdomen? Your face? Once you've identified where in the body you experience sadness, open your eyes and jot down a few notes about it. How does it differ from your physical experience of anger?

4. Again, sit comfortably with your eyes closed and spend a few minutes meditating. Allow yourself to fully relax before continuing. When you're ready, recall a time when you were afraid, and spend about five minutes reexperiencing the incident. Do a scan and notice how your body responds. Which areas of your body feel activated? Notice any reac-

tions—tight muscles, increased heartbeat, fluttering belly? Once you've identified where in the body you experience fear, open your eyes and jot down a few notes about it. How does it differ from your physical experience of sadness and anger?

5. Sit again with your eyes closed and spend a few minutes meditating. Once you're relaxed and settled, think of a specific time when you were truly joyful, and let yourself reexperience it. Recall all the details—the setting, who else was there (if anyone), everything you can. Do a scan and notice how your body feels. Are there any changes in your face? Your chest or abdomen? Does your posture change? Do you feel lighter? Once you've identified where in the body you experience joy, open your eyes and jot down a few notes about it. How does it differ from your physical experience of sadness, anger, and fear?

Knowing which physical cues correspond to which emotions will help you in recognizing your feelings, whether you're experiencing the primary emotions described above (anger, sadness, fear, or joy) or more complex emotions, such as anxiety (which is similar to fear but is generated through thoughts). Once you're able to recognize your emotions, you can begin to learn from them. Start focusing on emotional awareness in your daily meditation practice, and start a food-and-feelings journal (see the exercise and sample below) to begin building your awareness. If you still have trouble identifying emotions after trying the exercise above several times, see "Feeling? What Feeling?" below. People who are overweight and do a lot of emotional eating are more likely to have a hard time identifying their feelings—what psychologists call alexithymia.

Exercise: Track Your Food and Feelings

To start connecting the dots between your emotions and your eating behavior, keep your journal with you and record how you're feeling before and after eating, as in the sample chart below. For now, don't try to alter your behavior; just notice it, and keep your non-judgment cap on.

Time	What Emotion I Felt Before Eating	What I Ate	Was I Hungry?	What Emotion I Felt After Eating
10 A.M.	Fear about finishing report	Donuts	No	Guilty
Noon	Relief that I finished the report	Turkey sandwich and salad	Yes	Content
7 P.M.	Frustration that husband not home yet	An enormous bowl of pasta	Yes, but I kept eating long past fullness	Shame and anger
10 P.M.	Boredom; all TV shows are reruns	Chocolate chip cookies	No	Hopeless

Feeling? What Feeling?

If you remain stumped about what you're feeling after trying the "Mapping Your Emotions" exercise above, look at the chart below. With practice, you can use your body to access your emotions. Eventually, you'll be able to recognize the emotions directly.

Sensation	Might Signal	True Need
fluttering in upper chest	fear	safety, comfort
fluttering in upper chest	anxiety	relaxation
fatigue	boredom	stimulation
fatigue	sadness	connection
fatigue	tiredness	sleep
heat in the face	anger	reinstate a boundary
heat in the face	embarrassment	reassurance
heart racing	fear	safety
heart racing	anger	reinstate a boundary
heaviness in chest	loneliness	connection
jittery stomach	nervousness	relaxation

The Stress-and-Eating Cycle

To understand the dynamics of comfort eating, we also need to step back and look at the bigger picture: stress and its effects on our behavior. Emotions are part of this picture, but there is more. Stress undermines healthy habits, including healthy eating, weight loss, and overall health in dozens of ways, from altering the biochemistry of your very cells to making you less likely to exercise or plan and cook healthy meals. Among the most pervasive effects of stress are its effects on your moment-to-moment decision-making and almost automatic behavior—what psychologists call **stress reactivity**.

Most of us refer to stress daily—as in "I'm so stressed!"—but we rarely stop to think about what that means, let alone how stress affects us or how to manage it. One way to think of stress is that it's the experience we have when we perceive a threat to our health, happiness, or goals. Notice the word *perceive*—the fact is that our experience of stress is based on our perception, whether or not there's a real threat. That threat may come from the outside (a speeding taxi hurtling toward us, an impending deadline, a 3-year-old having a tantrum) or the inside (a thought such as "I'm always going to be overweight!" or an emotion like frustration or despair). In the swirl of daily life, dozens of daily factors give rise to stress: work, intimate relationships, traffic, money, parents, children, health problems, to-do lists, weather, loss, politics—the list goes on and on.

When we're too stressed, we naturally react—physically, mentally, emotionally, and behaviorally. Physically, our hearts pump faster, certain blood vessels constrict, and stored energy (in the form of sugar and fats) flows into our blood—all vestiges of our ancient fight-or-flight response that's designed to protect us from real danger. With chronic stress, our thoughts tend to speed up or become scattered or distorted, and often we have difficulty concentrating and making simple decisions. Emotionally, we often lock into negative feelings like fear or anger—or sometimes we feel numb. The experience of stress creates internal pressure that seems to demand a response. We feel like we have to *do something now* to ease the tension.

That's where our behavior comes in, and in particular, our "automatic pilot" behaviors. There are dozens of ways to cope with stress, but by adulthood it's common to come to rely on just a few. They become automatically linked with stress, and, whether or not they are healthy, they serve as coping mechanisms. Without judging, consider the simple facts of how people commonly cope with stress:

- Drink alcohol
- Smoke
- Take drugs (prescription, over-the-counter, or recreational)
- Go shopping

- Zone out in front of the TV
- Distract oneself by surfing the Internet
- Snap at one's spouse or children
- Withdraw socially
- Call a friend to vent
- Exercise, such as walking or jogging
- Exercise too much, to the point of exhaustion
- Avoid exercise
- Do yoga or meditate
- Eat food that's high in sugar, carbohydrates, or fat

Psychologists distinguish between **adaptive** and **maladaptive** coping strategies. Adaptive habits often involve a pause, some reflection, and consciously ingrained patterns of healthy behavior—e.g., "Wow, that confrontation with a neighbor was really stressful. A walk would help me blow off steam right now." Maladaptive habits, including chronic comfort eating (along with excessive drinking, smoking, and snapping at your spouse), often happen in a flash. They're automatic reactions that have been so "overlearned" that they're almost like a reflex. The diagram on the next page illustrates how stress-related eating can keep us trapped in a destructive cycle.

Stress and Automatic Eating

The following eating behaviors are common reactions to stress. Place a check mark next to those that look familiar to you.

Grabbing whatever food is available, which is often unhealthy	❑
Snacking between meals or grazing throughout the day	❑
Grabbing high-sugar, high-fat, high-salt processed foods	❑
Drinking more caffeine	❑
Drinking alcohol	❑
Skipping meals and overcompensating later	❑

Eating excessively large portions ❑
Bingeing (eating excessively large amounts of food in a very
    short period of time and feeling out of control) ❑
Eating for entertainment or other non-hunger reasons ❑
Not paying attention to the body's subtle signals of hunger ❑
Not paying attention to the body's subtle signals of fullness ❑

The Stress & Eating Cycle

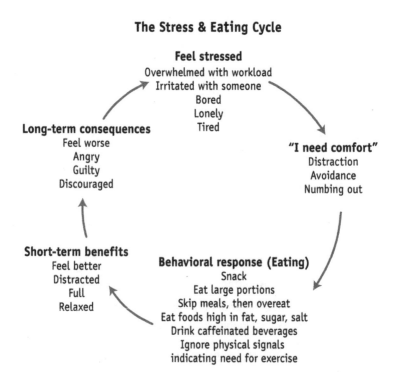

Feel stressed
Overwhelmed with workload
Irritated with someone
Bored
Lonely
Tired

"I need comfort"
Distraction
Avoidance
Numbing out

Long-term consequences
Feel worse
Angry
Guilty
Discouraged

Short-term benefits
Feel better
Distracted
Full
Relaxed

Behavioral response (Eating)
Snack
Eat large portions
Skip meals, then overeat
Eat foods high in fat, sugar, salt
Drink caffeinated beverages
Ignore physical signals
indicating need for exercise

Your Stress Profile

As you can see in the diagram above, we respond to stress on multiple
levels: thoughts, physical sensations, emotions, and behavior. Everyone's
response is unique. You can think of the bundle of sensations, thoughts,

emotions, and behaviors that kick in when you're stressed as your **stress profile.** In the exercise below, consider what happens when you are feeling stressed. Include food-related reactions and other types of behavior. If negative judgments come up, remember that removing the judgment we have about our bad habits lets us examine and understand them. Only then can we change them, if we decide to do so.

Exercise: What's Your Stress Profile?

To get to know your stress profile, it helps to think of a recent example, so remember a time that you were fairly stressed. Choose a moderately upsetting event, not an extremely upsetting one; intense stress can elicit different responses. List the stressful event or challenge below or in your journal. Then, using your mindfulness skills, describe the corresponding sensations, thoughts, and emotions you experienced, along with what you did (behavior), by giving a brief description in each column.

In the behavior column, include food-related reactions and other types of behavior. Also include activities that you *stopped* doing. For instance, during the stressful event, you might have stopped eating breakfast, stopped planning meals in advance, stopped exercising, or stopped calling your sister on Fridays to talk about your week.

Example: Meeting at which a colleague took credit for my work

Sensations	Thoughts	Emotions	Behavior
Tight jaw Eventual headache	I can't believe my colleague just said that! Focus on negative	Frustration Irritation Dread	Avoided colleague Skipped exercise Went out to dinner, ordered wine

Stressor, event, or challenge: _____

_____

Sensations	Thoughts	Emotions	Behavior

When you listed how you reacted behaviorally, did any part of your automatic stress response surprise you? Did your reaction affect your eating or physical activity? What did you learn about yourself? It's helpful to revisit this process multiple times with different stressors. Don't judge; just observe what happens inside of you with curiosity and kindness.

Now that you've begun to identify the pieces of your own stress profile, you can start practicing unpacking this bundle—in particular, when you find yourself eating unhealthy foods or avoiding physical activity. As always, the first goal is deep awareness without judgment. Without trying to do anything differently, just start asking yourself questions: What's happening in my body? What am I thinking? What am I feeling emotionally? And then, what do I end up doing? Learning to identify and separate the various parts of this "reactivity package" is the core of developing your abilities to change your patterns.

The High Cost of Chronic Stress

Human beings have always experienced stress, and our bodies are designed to deal with it. In every culture throughout history, life has presented a series of problems to be solved. The challenges change, but there have always been—and always will be—challenges. And as much as we might fantasize about a stress-free existence, that's not only impossible, it's not even desirable. A certain amount of stress motivates us to act, to finish projects, to find solutions, and to make important changes. Most of our accomplishments—raising children, reaching career goals, running a race—are accompanied by a certain amount of stress. Normal, healthy stress helps us accomplish things and propels us forward. What's unique about contemporary American culture is the *quantity* and *quality* of stress in our lives. Chronic stress has left us exhausted but simultaneously unable to relax—a state that many health experts call "tired but wired."

Our bodies and minds were designed to cope with intense, occasional *physical* stress—running from danger, for example. Our fight-or-flight response is an efficient, effective, automatic system for dealing with such acute challenges: your body's sympathetic nervous system churns out hormones such as adrenaline, which raises your heart rate and blood pressure to equip you to run.

While we may not face the life-threatening dangers of our ancestors, we increasingly have an accumulation of small and medium stressors—mostly psychological—and no release valve. Our nervous systems were *not* designed to deal with these unrelenting mental challenges, nor were they designed to manage the constant and often overwhelming stimulation that characterizes everyday life for many of us. We are encouraged to do more, accomplish more, and consume more—with very little ostensible incentive to relax, slow down, or replenish ourselves. Most of us juggle an overflow of commitments at work and at home and never feel we have enough time—and we assume that this is what life is all about and that we can and should balance it all (doesn't everyone?).

In fact, no culture in history has lived this way. Physiologically, chronic stress throws our stress response into overdrive, with the adrenal glands producing more adrenaline and cortisol.

Our bodies also have a mechanism that allows us to relax deeply, get restorative sleep, and recover from acute stress—the relaxation response. But unlike our body's stress response, the relaxation response is not automatic. Simultaneously, we have fewer built-in opportunities to use it. In fact, unless you consciously work to create the relaxation response in your own body, it's unlikely that you'll experience it with any frequency or regularity. One sign of our relaxation deficiency: more than 40 percent of Americans report difficulty sleeping due to stress.

The stakes are high. Chronic stress compromises metabolism and immune system function, increases our risk of overeating and other behaviors that harm our health, and ups our risk of heart disease, cancer, depression, and many other chronic illnesses. By some estimates, 60 to 80 percent of medical issues are triggered or made worse by stress.

Healthy Stress versus Unhealthy Stress

Healthy	Unhealthy
Occasional	Constant
Time-limited	Chronic
Motivating	Debilitating
Energizing	Depleting
Balanced by relaxation	Relentless
Consciously attended to	Unconsciously ignored
No long-term health consequences	Increased risk of many chronic illnesses

What the Science Says: Stress, Hormones, and Belly Fat

Research shows that there's a relationship between chronic stress, hunger and fullness hormones, inflammation, and abdominal fat. We know that chronic stress—as opposed to periodic stress—causes our bodies to produce higher amounts of hormones such as cortisol, which in turn leads the body to store more intra-abdominal fat. Whereas scientists long believed fat to be inert fuel storage for the body—not actively producing chemicals that impact other body systems—we now know that certain types of fat are not inert, but active, responding to and even producing hormones and inflammatory compounds. Intra-abdominal fat appears to be especially hormonally active, and evidence suggests that it may negatively alter levels of leptin and ghrelin, the hunger and fullness hormones, leading those with belly fat to feel hungry more often and have a harder time feeling full. It's a self-perpetuating cycle on the level of pure chemistry.

While not all aspects of the processes are clear yet, there is an apparent cycle of stress, accumulation of belly fat, and hormone imbalance that, once at a particular level, has a life of its own. This may help explain the physiological challenges that overweight people have in shedding pounds—and it's further evidence of the damaging effects of chronic stress on our health.

Fortunately, people are not doomed by their biology. Eating more mindfully and slowly reregulates hormone levels. One study, for instance, showed that eating slowly can shift the levels of PYY, a hormone that helps people feel full. Another study showed that overweight women who practiced mindfulness reduced their levels of cortisol and their abdominal fat. And many studies now show that practicing mindfulness lowers stress.

The Cost of Constant Connection

The sensory stimulation we're exposed to has ramped up over the last few decades to the point of overload. The deluge of information, imagery, and sounds on television, computers, tablets, and smartphones—and the expectation that people are constantly available through instant messaging and the like—is unprecedented.

Downtime and meaningful *social* connection is increasingly trumped by compulsive *digital* connection. For a lot of people, what were once brief interludes of relaxation are now spent checking email, searching online, or texting. That means more stimulation, less relaxation, less sleep, and more stress reactivity—all of which can increase unhealthy eating habits. More and more, we are "tired but wired," and it's very difficult to maintain healthy habits in that state.

Besides eroding our downtime, being constantly connected adds to our stress level in other ways, by multiplying our choices and increasing the extent to which we compare ourselves with others. Whereas we once thought about how we "measure up" compared with our immediate community, we now judge ourselves against the whole world: How's my cooking compared with that foodie-blog superstar's? How's my portfolio looking compared with Warren Buffett's? How's my body looking compared with Brooklyn Decker's? These comparisons—enabled by the Internet and social media—often happen subconsciously, but they take an enormous toll on our self-esteem and increase our stress levels. Our brains and bodies are not equipped to process the level of stimulation they receive without respite. In fact, we are training our brains to have limited attention spans and poor memory—and to accept highly disrupted lives.

The hyperstimulation and distraction that have become the norm are the antithesis of mindfulness. But given that the Internet and cell phones aren't going anywhere, it's up to you to take a step back and see how your connectivity may be affecting your stress levels, your habits, and your health.

Choices: A Blessing or a Curse?

We value abundance and choice in this country, but how does choice impact our stress levels? These days we're prone to "choice overload," the phenomenon of having so many options at every turn that we spend great quantities of time *deciding*. Everyone can relate: You go to the grocery store to buy peanut butter and find no fewer than twenty-five types to choose from. Or you want to buy something relatively straightforward—say, a blender—and decide to buy online to save time, then find yourself wading through hundreds of blenders on various websites, comparing features and prices and reading dozens of reviews. We rarely stop and think about it, but choice—a good thing, in theory—can be very stressful. Our brains weren't designed to be constantly filtering this level of fairly useless information, making comparisons, and pressuring ourselves to make the *best* choice, rather than a *good* choice. Like other stressors, the plethora of choices we confront in our daily lives keeps our brain "on" and further erodes opportunities for relaxation. Worse still, it makes food choices much more complicated. Interestingly, in Chinese medicine, having too many choices is said to contribute to an imbalance known as "liver qi stagnation," a common diagnosis among Americans that can lead to insomnia and irritability.

The Chemistry of Comfort Eating

Why is it that when you're angry, anxious, lonely, scared, or stressed, a few bites of ice cream, mashed potatoes, or chocolate can soothe your nerves and make you feel better? Part of it is pure association, the way humans learn. If your mom or grandmother baked a lot of cookies when you were a child and you have positive memories of that, you probably crave cookies when you're in need of comfort now. Or it might be curried chicken for you, or garlic mashed potatoes, or chocolate cream pie. These memories are stored in your brain, in an area called the mammillary body within your hypothalamus. Research has shown that childhood patterns are powerful factors in adult eating behavior.

Still, people don't generally eat cauliflower or lentils for comfort, even if they were served these foods as a child. Classic comfort foods are high in calories and fat, sugar, or salt—think macaroni and cheese, lasagna, cobbler, ice cream, cookies, or chocolate. This is no accident. When we engage in emotional or stress-related eating, part of what's going on is that on a chemical level, our brains and bodies are trying to self-regulate. Our brains and bodies are continually seeking balance—homeostasis—and in a given moment, overeating carbohydrate- and fat-laden foods is one way to achieve this.

How we feel emotionally in a given moment or on a given day is determined in part by the levels of natural chemicals in our brain called neurotransmitters. There are several that influence our mood. One of these is a well-researched neurotransmitter called serotonin, which has a direct link with appetite and food. The mechanisms are complex and still being studied, but essentially, when we are adequately producing serotonin and our brains are using it well, we feel happy, optimistic, and upbeat—and our appetite is diminished. When our brains are not using serotonin well, we feel sad, pessimistic, or irritable—and we tend to crave food. It's not about the *amount* of serotonin but about how the brain is regulated by it and regulates it. Depression and some anxiety disorders are associated with the brain's inadequate use of serotonin, though scientists don't yet understand the mechanisms. And guess what nutrient can flip the serotonin switch to increase its availability? Carbohydrates—the primary component of most comfort foods. Dietary fat, another common component, triggers the release of dopamine, a neurotransmitter that regulates our capacity to experience rewards and feel pleasure.

It's no exaggeration to say that some people self-medicate with food much as others self-medicate with alcohol or drugs—and get stuck in similarly addictive patterns. (Not that the two issues are mutually exclusive—many people do both.) Studies have shown that carbohydrates affect the brain's neurotransmitters in a manner similar to nicotine, and animal studies have noted similarities between eating a fatty diet and cocaine addiction.

Caffeine + Stress = More Stress

Millions of Americans, some 90 percent, drink caffeinated beverages on a daily basis. People drink coffee, tea, and caffeinated soda to jump-start their day, as an afternoon "pick-me-up," or when they need to focus. For a lot of people, it's a comforting ritual. But when it comes to stress levels, caffeine may be making things worse. Researchers have shown that caffeine amplifies your body's stress response, both physically and psychologically, and that its effects in the body last much longer than previously thought. In a double-blind, placebo-controlled study, scientists at Duke University studied the effects of caffeine on several dozen habitual coffee drinkers. They found that caffeine, consumed in the morning and at lunchtime, raised participants' blood pressure and stress-hormone levels throughout the day and into the evening. What's more, when people experienced an ordinary stressful event, caffeine exaggerated both the body's stress response and the psychological *perception* of stress. In other words, caffeine can aggravate the already damaging effects of stress on our bodies and our moods. Additional studies have echoed these results and shown that habitual caffeine use saps energy and worsens insomnia. It can be a vicious cycle, since the more tired you feel, the more likely you are to reach for coffee or tea—which ultimately further saps your energy. If you're experiencing a lot of stress, fatigue, or both, consider cutting down or eliminating caffeine while adding in something that lowers your stress level, like regular exercise or yoga. But do so gradually; caffeine withdrawal can leave you dragging and with a bad headache.

People who experience chronic stress may be especially prone to comfort eating. As we've discussed, chronic stress makes our bodies churn out high levels of stress hormones such as cortisol, without the corresponding balancing relaxation response (in which stress hormones naturally drop). Cortisol stimulates our appetites and makes us more likely to choose foods that are high in sugar and/or fat. One recent study of women suggested that those who have chronic high stress report engaging in "comfort eating" more often than those who have lower stress levels—and, not surprisingly, the stressed comfort eaters have higher amounts of harmful abdominal fat.

Compared with coping mechanisms such as alcohol and illegal drug use, comfort eating is safer in the most immediate sense, more socially acceptable, and legal—but it is damaging and not sustainable long-term without its own consequences. While comfort eating can lead to a quick mood improvement from the rise in serotonin, the effects are temporary, and it can lead to a hormonal roller-coaster ride that ends up *increasing* your stress levels. When you ingest simple carbohydrates, your blood sugar shoots up and subsequently crashes down. This crash increases your stress-hormone levels, which makes you crave more of the same high-carb foods. Over time, especially when combined with a sedentary lifestyle, that pattern decreases your ability to adapt to stress and can lead to weight gain, insulin resistance, and chronic illness.

Knowing the biology of mood and food can help to loosen the grip of judgment and shame that often accompany overeating and can also help you understand why willpower alone is not enough. Understanding what's happening biochemically can also help you make wiser choices to self-regulate. Getting regular exercise and sufficient sleep, increasing your exposure to sunlight during the day, and eating healthy meals that contain both protein and slow-burning carbohydrates (such as whole grains and vegetables) may help to balance your levels of serotonin, dopamine, and other neurotransmitters. In addition, support your behavior by creating environments that help you make better choices: kitchens set up to facilitate healthy cooking, healthy snack options planned and available, bedrooms that are conducive to sleep, sneakers always in the car for spontaneous walks, and regular daily relaxation activities to lower your stress level. Using your mindfulness skills changes your experience of stress—by tuning in to your body's signals, your thoughts, and your emotions, you can figure out your true needs.

Insights and Inspirations: Sharon, age 30

When I feel a strong negative feeling, it terrifies me, in part I think because I grew up with a mom who was highly emotional and had a bad temper. She seemed to always be on the verge of losing it, and the less I set her off, the better. I've kept my feelings very contained for most of my life, which turns out to not be such a good strategy for adult relationships. I feel like I have low-level anxiety all the time, and I keep it at bay with constant snacking.

Balancing Your Stress Cup

Think of your stress level as liquid in a cup. We're at our healthiest when it's no more than moderately full at some points during the day, and mostly empty at others. We need enough intermittent stimulation and "healthy stress" to keep us motivated, engaged, and growing, but not so much that the cup is overflowing. Nonetheless, for many of us, the cup overflows not occasionally but *continually*. And many never empty the cup, certainly not on a daily basis.

Keeping your stress cup balanced—breaking free from the chronic-stress cycle—is one of the most important things you can do to take charge of your health and improve your eating habits. Reducing the stress in your cup does not mean you need to go on a monthlong retreat from your life. In fact, building in restorative time *on a daily basis* and incorporating it into your everyday life is more beneficial than occasional long bouts of downtime. Your daily meditation practice is an essential foundation, but it's crucial to find other ways to slow down, relax, and take care of your body. Yoga and stretching have been shown to induce the relaxation response. Physical affection, regular or moderate to intense exercise, social support, and genuine laughter can all help to lower your stress levels.

Intention plays a huge role here, because our cultural default is debilitating stress. Start with the journal exercise below.

Exercise: Getting Ready to Stress Less

Spend some time thinking honestly about what a less stressful life would look and feel like. Think about what you would gain (e.g., improved health and happiness, better sleep) and also what you would lose (e.g., missing out on fun, always knowing what's going on with your loved ones and in the world). Do the benefits outweigh the losses? Are you willing to make a commitment to reduce the stress in your life? Think of several specific things you could do to rebalance your life or lower your stress—for example, cancel an extraneous meeting, make a date to meet a friend for a walk, or go to the movies with your spouse. Revisit the section on goals for sustainable change (page 58) and create goals related to stress reduction.

Optimal goal:
Desirable goal:
Minimal goal:
Behavior to track:

~

When Amy, age 34, came to one of our programs, she had been trying to kick her habit of eating baked goods at work. Like many offices, hers was rife with cookies, muffins, donuts, and candy. And while this kind of environment alone makes healthy eating challenging, together we realized that for Amy, the biggest culprit wasn't muffins and scones, but chronic stress. A marketing VP, she had long prided herself on working long and hard hours, often taking her laptop or smartphone into bed with her and catching up on work emails until midnight. "I had managed to convince myself that I only needed four or five hours of sleep a night. I woke up alert and ready to go. I told myself I was doing fine," she says. At some point, though, she started to feel exhausted mid-morning. She compensated for that by eating baked goods or sweets every few hours, usually washing them down with a cup of coffee. Not surprisingly, she gained weight—mostly in her abdomen—and her insulin and triglyceride levels began to climb into the danger zone. Willing herself to choose healthier foods wasn't working, however.

Once she started working with us, she realized that nothing was going to change until she tackled the root cause, chronic stress. She says, "I started with one little thing: not bringing my tablet or my smartphone to bed. God, that was the hardest part. Sometimes I'd jump out of bed to get one of them." Focusing on one change at a time with the help of sustainable goals, she began the process of reducing stress. Six months later, she had put boundaries on her work hours, had cut down to one cup of coffee in the morning, and had started a walking routine with a friend in the neighborhood. She was sleeping longer and more deeply, and most of the time was able to resist sweets in the office. "I didn't crave them in the same way," she says.

Paying close attention to the choices you make every day and looking at the bigger picture of your life are helpful steps in reducing chronic stress. Evaluating your life doesn't mean avoiding every stressor or going to live off the grid in a forest somewhere.

Every so often, revisit your Wheel of Health and see which areas you're functioning well in and which need more balance. Are there areas where you can cut back? Be especially careful when considering adding to what's "on your plate," whether that's caring for your grandson on an overfull day or agreeing to join the board of a nonprofit you care about. It's not that you need to say no to everything, but it's important to ask yourself where the time for new commitments will come from, what meaning they will bring you, and how you'll balance any additions to your stress cup. When it comes to life balance and your stress levels, try to shift from general activity and "busy-ness" to carefully chosen, meaningful engagement. Regular meditation will support this process.

CHAPTER 8

A Body to Love

"Your body is precious.
It is our vehicle for awakening.
Treat it with care."

—Buddha

When you look in a full-length mirror, what's the first thing that happens? Do you relax and smile, warm eyes taking in the person in front of you, the way you would greet a close friend or a loved one? Or do your stiffen and brace yourself, eyes hardening to a narrow focus as a harsh inner voice details all your flaws? Or perhaps you look only at your face, avoiding the body you would rather not think about or see. Or, like many people who struggle with their weight, maybe you just look away as soon as possible.

How we view our bodies and what we tell ourselves about them can greatly influence the way we eat. In our work with clients at Duke IM, we see how constant self-criticism and low self-esteem can undermine efforts to create lasting change. For example, if a glance in the mirror sets off a litany of putdowns—*you're ugly, you're fat, no partner would ever want you*—you may find yourself depressed and hopeless and looking for chocolate, a spiral that can lead to more negative thoughts and more emotional eating.

Body image is a complicated issue for people who are trying to lose weight and change their habits. For some it can seem wrong, or even unhealthy, to develop a positive body image before losing weight. If you let yourself feel good about your appearance now, the thinking goes, how will you ever motivate yourself to change? But that thinking is a trap that keeps you stuck in unhealthy patterns.

Letting Go of Your Inner Critic

Karen, age 39, gained 30 pounds after having her first child and three years later hadn't been able to take it off. Whereas she once enjoyed clothes shopping, she now dreaded going into stores. Her stomach, which had lost its tone and was covered with stretch marks, made her especially uncomfortable, and she avoided looking at it. When she did catch her image in the mirror, she felt disgusted and told herself she was a weak person who had clearly let herself go. At night, sad and exhausted, she would often reach for her go-to comfort food: oatmeal-raisin cookies. After three years of beating up on herself, Karen could see that her harsh Inner Critic wasn't helping, but, at the same time, it seemed self-deceptive to feign positive feelings about a body she didn't want. Wasn't she supposed to feel good about herself *after* she lost a few pounds?

Like many women who want to lose weight, Karen equated criticizing her body—often with judgmental words like "disgusting" and "slob"—with self-control. If you can just keep enough pressure on yourself, the reasoning goes, you can change the way you eat. It's an easy mind-set to fall into, and as we discussed in earlier chapters, a pattern of thinking that the diet industry and American media encourage. But here's the problem: it doesn't work.

Think of it this way: If you had a loved one you were trying to help, would you scream insults at her? Would you greet her with disgust, list her faults, berate her, and call her gross and hopeless? Would you let someone treat your best friend or a colleague that way? Of course not. And yet, we aim this kind of talk inward and call it self-discipline. In actual fact, it's the Inner Critic. This harsh, insidious voice—with its distorted perspective—*gets in the way* of true progress and discipline.

An essential key to changing your eating habits is learning to tune in to your body's messages, to recognize and respond to the cues that tell you when you're hungry and when you've had enough. But in order to listen to your body, you have to be able to physically feel those cues; you can't learn from sensations you don't allow yourself to experience. We have seen again and again that people can listen to their bodies, and respond to the messages their bodies communicate, only when they've accepted their physical selves enough to truly *inhabit* them.

People who struggle with their weight often live "from the neck up," judging their bodies with harsh thoughts instead of experiencing and feeling them. Our bodies are amazing sources of information, but in order to access that wisdom, we have to connect with them, which means letting go of the Inner Critic. That's all well and good, you may say, but how is it possible to be nonjudgmental and accepting of something you want to change? The key to reconciling these two seemingly contradictory ideas—the need for acceptance and the desire for change—is mindful compassion.

Imagine what might happen if you were to stop for a moment and just look at yourself in the mirror for thirty seconds. During this time, you don't judge, or assess, or denigrate, or even plan for improvements in the future. You simply are present in the moment and look. *Those are my arms. That is what my stomach looks like. Those are my eyes. That is a whole person looking back at me, and this is what she looks like.* If a voice inside starts hurling insults or making a list of all the things that are wrong, just notice those thoughts, label them as "judgments," and refocus your attention on describing what you see: descriptive but not judgmental. Continue looking. That is mindfulness—just gently being in the moment with the person you are.

Now, what if you could look at your reflection without demanding perfection? What if you could see the flaws without judging them, and just observe? Perhaps you see a soft belly or a belly sloping down. Just describe what you see without judgmental words. Ask yourself, "Would it be possible to treat this body with kindness and appreciation for all it does for me, even though it isn't perfect, and even though I am working to make it healthier?" Imagine wrapping your body in compassion and what that might feel like. How might it change the decisions you make for the rest of the day?

Insights and Inspirations: Nicole, age 38

I love the idea of being nonjudgmental and kind to myself, but I find it almost impossible to do in certain situations. I went bathing suit shopping the other day. As I walked into the store, I told myself I wasn't going to put myself down when I tried on suits. But then I was looking through the sale rack and they didn't have anything in my size, only much smaller options. Before I knew it, I was going off on myself again. Why did you have dessert the other night? You're so weak. You've totally lost control. You'll always be fat and UGLY. And on and on. I hadn't even found a suit to try on yet and I was already miserable.

For many of us, negative thoughts and feelings about our bodies are a deeply ingrained habit—another "packaged response" that we have come to accept as normal. Even when we know intellectually that we want to change, the Inner Critic voice can show up as an automatic reflex in certain situations. Before we even realize it, we are judging ourselves. We try on a dress and we look for flaws. We walk into a party and compare ourselves unfavorably to the prettiest woman in the room. Even receiving compliments can be uncomfortable, triggering an immediate "Yes, but . . ." response. We need to learn to recognize and eventually drop the negative body judgment from our thinking. Instead, we need to learn to *experience* the body rather than *thinking about* it.

Your Mindfulness Toolkit

We're adding new tools to your mindfulness toolkit. In addition to the practices from earlier chapters, in this chapter you'll learn another exercise to expand your awareness and create the ground-work for healthy choices.

- Healing Self-Touch

Building Mindful Compassion

A mindful approach to body image can help us explore, in a nonjudg-mental way, what we've been telling ourselves. This increased awareness is the first step toward undoing a packaged response.

Exercise: Body Image Awareness

Try this exercise to consider what kinds of beliefs you have about yourself and how they affect you. John Tarrant, Ph.D., a dear col-league, Zen Roshi, and writer inspired this exercise through his meditation teachings over the years. To gain additional practice, see the work of Byron Katie.

When you look in the mirror, what do you tell yourself?

_____

_____

When someone gives you a compliment, how do you feel? What do you tell yourself? How do you react? Do you look the person in the eye and say thank you? Do you contradict the person either out loud or silently to yourself?

_____

_____

_____

_____

_____

Do a brief Body Scan and notice your thoughts about each body part as it is scanned. What are your beliefs about yourself and your body as you bring awareness to different parts?

_____

_____

_____

_____

Now consider these self-statements and beliefs. Ask if they are helping or hurting you.

Pick one of the statements and then ask yourself the following questions:

- How do I treat myself when I believe this?
- How do I treat others when I believe this?
- How does this statement impact my desire to take better care of myself?
- How does this statement help me feel empowered to take better care of myself?
- How does this statement affect my ability to meet my short- and long-term goals?
- What would it be like not to hold this belief?

Remember that undoing a packaged response takes time, intention, and practice. It's not a quick or easy process, especially when the self-criticism habit may have been years in the making.

Sometimes it's a specific physical change—the weight gain after childbirth, or the thick hips that arrive after spending a couple of years in a stressful job, or the gray hair and lined face of menopause—that starts the cycle of negative thoughts about our bodies. But often the pattern of self-denigration, or at least the seeds of it, goes back decades. In our culture, learning to focus on physical imperfections is often part of growing up, and it starts far younger than you might think. In one study, children as young as 3 years old identified larger bodies negatively and thinner bodies positively. Researchers found that they had picked up their moms' own body images and attitudes about weight—"fat" is bad and "skinny" is good.

Insights and Inspirations: Lori, age 51

I still remember sitting on my parents' bed as a child and listening to my mother put herself down as she would get ready for parties. She'd try on one dress after another, sucking in her stomach and saying things like "My legs are so short and stubby," and sighing. She was thin and beautiful! She hated her hair, and she'd flip it around, calling it hopeless and mousy brown and flat. I loved fastening my mom's necklace and handling her makeup. Once I remarked how beautiful she looked, and she leaned into the mirror and traced her fingers over the fine lines around her eyes. "I wish," she said. After she'd leave, I'd play dress-up. I would zip into one of her dresses and try on her jewelry. Then I'd stand in front of the mirror and suck in my stomach and study my face for blemishes.

Many women can recall some variation of these scenes from their childhood. As teenagers, the self-criticism often ramps up. Allie described to us the intimate, often bonding moments women share that center around criticizing one body part after another. She and her friends would pore over articles in teen magazines looking for the one secret that would make them more attractive and therefore, in their minds, more popular. The stories would give advice on how to choose a prom dress that best hides problem areas, or what to wear if you hate your stomach, your butt, or your thighs. At sleepovers, they would rank the pretty girls in their school by feature: best eyes, best breasts, best hair, et cetera, all the while discussing their own shortcomings.

Over the years, this harsh Inner Critic can become an unconscious but deeply ingrained habit, one that guides your eyes to every "ugly" feature and runs an immediate tally of all the ways you fall short of some idealized perfection. In today's media-saturated environment, you don't have to look far for unattainable ideals: sculpted sports stars, Photoshopped cover models, surgically enhanced celebrities. The images are everywhere. But compare yourself to every Internet pop-up ad, magazine cover, and billboard that you pass, and you could fall short of a dozen impossible standards before you get to work in the morning.

The Problem with Perfection

Whether we look in the mirror and compare ourselves to some impossible ideal (the beach volleyball star with washboard abs) or even to our own healthy goals (say, a stronger, more toned version of our current self), *we never measure up*. When we expect perfection, we are always disappointed. And that disappointment, along with the self-criticism and the low self-esteem that go with it, can become a downward spiral that undermines our eating habits and our health.

Research tells us that people who are successful at maintaining weight loss give themselves permission to be imperfect. Again, that doesn't mean you have to force a false sense of happiness about the roll of fat you can pinch around your belly. Rather, think of permission to be imperfect as the freedom to *appreciate who you are* and to encourage your own progress through life, even when you fall short and make mistakes along the way.

Margaret, a 38-year-old engineer, had always hated her large thighs and, as a teenager and young adult, coveted her older sister's legs. "She always had those 'perfect' shapely thighs that didn't touch together," she says. Margaret had a YMCA membership but was embarrassed to go to exercise classes there and made excuses to avoid going to the beach with friends in the summer. But using mindfulness, she was able to start recognizing her Inner Critic for what it was—not truth, but judgment and meanness. She says, "One day I counted the insults. I called myself ugly or fat about thirty-five times." As she worked on non-judgment in meditation, it began to spill over into her life, and Body Scans helped her to start *experiencing* her body more, especially her thighs. "I stopped thinking about my thighs compared to my sister's or anybody else's," she says. "I stopped bashing my body." Instead, she tuned in to how her thighs felt throughout the day—as they enabled her to stand up and sit down, walk up and down stairs, play tag with her 6-year-old nephew, and many other things.

By actually *feeling* her thighs—experiencing them—she started to appreciate their power and strength, and this had a positive ripple effect. She started mountain-biking with friends on the weekends and taking spinning classes at the Y, which made her further appreciate what her body could do for her. The increased exercise made her feel better, both physically and emotionally, and seemed to help regulate her appetite. She also started eating more vegetables and stopped overeating routinely. "It was really pretty simple: I just felt better, and I wanted to *keep* feeling better," she recalls. "It's crazy to think about how much space that critical voice in my head occupied. It led me on such a downward spiral. It's not that I never hear it anymore, but I know how to recognize it and deal with it now. It doesn't have power over me."

Exercise: Embracing Imperfection

Remember when you rode a bike for the first time without training wheels? It was wobbly and touch-and-go. Remember the emotions—how free you felt, how independent, what an accomplishment that was. Now remember what you did when you fell off. You got back on and did it again until you could master the skill. In that moment, you gave yourself permission to be imperfect. It didn't make you lazy; it freed you to move forward because you weren't saddled down with feelings of failure and inadequacy.

How do you talk to yourself now when you make a mistake or don't measure up to an ideal? How do you talk to yourself when you look in the mirror and notice that you look tired, or that your belly is round, or that you have cellulite on your thighs? How do you talk to yourself when you step on a scale? How do you talk to yourself when you eat healthy food and exercise—and when you don't?

Can you imagine accepting your body just as it is? Can you imagine embracing your physical self, whether you lose weight, gain weight, or stay the same? Think of one behavior you'd like to change that would be healthy for your body. Can you envision yourself deciding to make this change, encouraging yourself along the way, accepting that you may not get it right all the time and deciding to move forward anyway? Can you imagine congratulating yourself when you are successful—but accepting your body and yourself regardless?

Reconnecting with Your Body

In order to develop healthy eating habits and increase our physical activity, we need to connect with our bodies. As we've described, our bodies are amazing sources of information. They can tell us when we're hungry, when we're full, when we're tired, thirsty, sore from a workout, or antsy because we have been sitting too long. When we learn to register the

Insights and Inspirations: Lydia, age 28

In high school, I always took a lot of pictures with my friends. I have whole scrapbooks filled with pictures of the good times we had. Then when I went to college, I gained a lot of weight. I only have a few pictures of myself from that time, and the truth is I hardly ever look at them. One thing I've tried to change as I reconnect with my body is getting comfortable looking at pictures of myself. I started with my phone. Whenever I had a moment of feeling good or happy, or even just a moment when I wasn't feeling bad about myself, I'd pull out my phone and snap a picture. Then I would look at the picture and see if I could see the person I was feeling inside. It took a while. At first looking at the pictures was hard. I had to work through some pretty bad feelings before I could just look at them calmly. But the more I practiced and looked at the pictures, the more I realized that I had no idea what I really look like. I started to see that I had moments when I was strong and happy, maybe even glowing, maybe even beautiful. It changed something inside me to be able to see myself this way. It had been so long since I'd felt anything but shame. I started to keep some of the pictures and look at them when I needed reassurance. I noticed that as I got more comfortable with the pictures, it also got easier to pay attention to when I was tired, or hungry or full. It was like I was no longer turning away from myself. A few weeks ago, I decided to send a picture of myself to a friend. It felt like a huge step. I never would have done that a few years ago.

signals and sensations our bodies give us, we can respond with care and kindness. *Ahhh, hungry—let me offer you something nourishing. Ahhh, full—let me stop eating now so you will be comfortable. Thirst? Here is water. Tired? How about a rest?* All compassionate responses—and all better and healthier than the have-some-potato-chips-and-shut-up attitude we can take when we are trying to pretend our bodies aren't there. But before we can fully meet our bodies' needs, we have to *know* what our bodies need—something that is difficult if we can't look at ourselves or listen to our sensations.

That's where improving our body image and letting go of the Inner Critic voice can make an important difference. **Constant self-criticism disconnects us from our bodies, making it nearly impossible to tune in and listen.** Over time, it's possible to become so focused on harsh judgments and external appearance that we live in our heads with little experience of our bodies at all. But learning to reconnect with your physical self—learning to feel or experience what is there and inhabit your body without judgment—can be hard, even painful. Like any relationship, it takes time and patience. Try the Healing Self-Touch exercise below, developed with Sasha Loring, M.Ed., L.C.S.W., to help you get started.

🔊 Mindfulness Tool: Healing Self-Touch

The following exercise is an opportunity to reconnect with your body and treat yourself with compassion, especially when you notice your harsh Inner Critic.

1. Begin with a relaxation exercise. Bring awareness to and relax each body area—feet, legs, abdomen, shoulders, arms, neck, and face.

2. Now, bring attention to your hands. Imagine that your hands are beginning to fill up with kindness, however you can envision that happening ... your hands are full of kindness, caring, warmth, and tenderness.

3. Place one hand over your heart. Notice your breathing. Feel the caring quality of your heart. Let it come through your

hands. Let all the mental chatter just come and go, coming back to a sense of tenderness and caring. Relax your hands.

4. Now lift one hand and place it on the opposite arm—a gentle, caring touch. After gently touching your arm, conveying tender care, gently drop your hand. Now lift the other hand and place it on the opposite arm—a kind and caring touch.

5. Just notice what this feels like, the sense of touching. What is your reaction? What is going through your mind? Notice, without judging, what thoughts come up . . . just touching with kindness.

6. Slowly move your hands to your abdomen. Let them rest and move with your abdomen as you breathe. Notice your reaction. Continue to feel the kindness in your hands, a sense of holding yourself in tenderness.

7. Next, move both your hands to your thighs. Gently place them wherever is comfortable, perhaps wondering if you can touch them with a sense of appreciation. Completely relax, allowing tenderness for all the feelings this may bring up.

8. Again, place one or both hands over your heart. Notice your breathing. Feel the caring quality of your heart. Let it come through your hands. Let all the mental chatter just come and go, coming back to a sense of tenderness and caring.

9. In the last moments of this process, you can continue to rest your hands where they are, or if you feel there is another part of your body that could use a tender, caring touch, move your hand there. Continue to rest with a sense of warmth toward yourself.

10. Slowly bring your attention back to the room. When you are finished with the exercise, take a few minutes to write in your journal. Consider what happened. What did you notice? What was difficult? What felt comfortable? What was helpful?

Insights and Inspirations: Liz, age 44

I hadn't gone to the doctor in four years. I'd been avoiding a physical because I dreaded seeing how much weight I'd gained. And I certainly didn't want to talk about it. I knew I needed to take care of myself better, but, for the most part, I just wanted to pretend the weight wasn't there. I knew that if I went to the doctor, I wouldn't be able to ignore it anymore. But doing the Healing Self-Touch exercise softened something in me. I felt compassion for myself, not criticism about the weight. I surveyed my friends the next day about their primary care doctors. I wanted to find someone who would reinforce the compassion, not the self-criticism. I made an appointment—the doctor was great, very caring. She tested my cholesterol and blood pressure—both were too high. We're doing regular check-ins to track my progress losing weight and getting my numbers down.

Honoring Your Body

When you start to listen to your body and honor it, your body responds. When you look at your body with compassion, you give yourself a chance to step out from under the burden of constant criticism. When you sense your body without judgment, it can be an opportunity to get information you need to improve your health—for example, what Liz learned about her weight, blood pressure, and cholesterol when she went to the doctor—without piling on the judgmental stories.

Revisit the "data versus story" exercise that you did on page 82. How might you apply this mindfulness technique to improving your body image? Read the following examples and come up with healthy responses to the data. Then think of a couple of examples from your own life and habits.

Exercise: Data versus Story—Body Image

Sample

Jumbled reaction: *I just walked into the party, and the room is filled with skinny women. I am probably the biggest woman here. Everyone else looks good in her dress.*

Story: *I look like an elephant in heels. No one will want to talk to me. I don't belong here.*

Data: *I am larger than most of the women in this room.*

Healthy response to data: *I am larger, and I am overweight. That's why I have begun to shift how I eat. Losing weight will take time and effort, but I am taking better care of myself.*

In the next two examples, the data has been separated from the story for you. See if you can come up with healthy responses using the data rather than the story.

1. Jumbled reaction: *A man just told me I look really nice in this color blue. I'm so uncomfortable that my stomach hurts.*

   Story: *I'm sure he just said that because it is the one nice thing you can say to someone of my size. I should make a self-deprecating joke.*

   Data: *Someone just gave me a compliment.*

   Healthy response to data: _____

   _____

   _____

   _____

   _____

2. Jumbled reaction: *I just tried on my favorite pants and they won't button. I've gained so much weight in the past six months, I am totally out of control.*

    Story: *I am gross and fat, and I will never look good again.*

    Data: *I've put on 20 pounds. My stomach is bigger and softer than it used to be.*

    Healthy response to data: _____

    _____

    _____

    _____

    _____

Now come up with a couple of examples from your own life. Parse the data from the story and then come up with a healthy response using the data rather than the story.

3. Jumbled reaction: _____

    _____

    _____

    Story: _____

    _____

    Data: _____

    _____

    Healthy response to data: _____

    _____

    _____

    _____

    _____

    _____

4. Jumbled reaction: _____

_____

_____

Story: _____

_____

Data: _____

_____

Healthy response to data: _____

_____

_____

_____

_____

Appreciating Your Body

Even when we aren't criticizing our bodies, we often take them for granted. This is natural, but when trying to heal your relationship with your body, appreciation and gratitude can go a long way (as in any relationship). Think about how much your body does for you. Your body carries you through your day. It fights off infection. It allows you to smell the flowers in a garden and see the smile on a child's face. Because of your body, you can taste your favorite foods, hold the hand of someone you love, cry when you are sad, and laugh when you are happy. When you tune in to it, your body can tell you much of what you need to know in order to be healthy. Even though it isn't perfect, it holds great wisdom. And it needs you. The time to embrace it and care for it isn't around the corner or when you've reached a certain goal—it's today.

Exercise: Gratitude Letter

Write a letter of appreciation and thanks to your body. Think about what your body has done for you today, what it's done for you this year, and what it's done your whole life. If you aren't sure what to say, start with these phrases:

I am grateful to you for . . .

_____

Without you, I wouldn't be able to . . .

_____

Thank you for giving me . . .

_____

I admire you because . . .

_____

I love you because . . .

_____

Read the letter after you have written it, then put it in an envelope and keep it in a safe place. Take the letter out and read it once a week for a month. If possible, choose a quiet place where you will have time to meditate, to watch your thoughts and feelings. Then notice how the letter affects your feelings. If there is a particular part of the body that you struggle with a lot, consider a letter just to that part, in addition to the more general one above.

Our relationship with our bodies, often invisible and unconscious, is a powerful factor in what, how, and why we eat—and in whether and how we exercise. In this chapter you've learned to use mindfulness to recognize and examine your current relationship and to begin shifting it. Recognizing the Inner Critic and separating it from description only—the story versus the data—is an important skill. It will help you learn to observe your body without judging it, and learn to feel and inhabit your body without thinking about it. By freeing yourself from the expectations of perfection—*I must wait until I'm perfect to feel good about myself and treat myself well*—you can begin to give yourself the compassionate, loving care you've always needed and deserved.

Realizing that your body is yours to care for—and treating it that way—will have positive ripple effects on your habits, your emotional well-being, and your overall health. For Margaret, recognizing her Inner Critic cleared the way for better eating and exercise habits. "It just became really simple. I felt good and wanted to keep feeling good," she said. Cultivating a positive, loving relationship with your body may be the ultimate in intrinsic motivation, setting you up for a lifetime of healthy eating.

CHAPTER 9

Know Your Triggers

"This being human is a guest house.
Every morning a new arrival.
A joy, a depression, a meanness,
some momentary awareness comes
as an unexpected visitor. . . .
Be grateful for whatever comes,
because each has been sent
as a guide from beyond."

—Rumi, "The Guest House"

B y now you've become more familiar with aspects of yourself and your life that can be difficult to look at—habits that are under-mining your health, imbalances in your life, your reactions to stress and difficult emotions. And as we've emphasized, mindful aware-ness is the foundation for lasting change. Awareness does not happen in a flash, and you can't just snap your fingers to produce mindfulness. Instead, it's a daily, moment-to-moment practice, a new framework for perception that makes it possible to counteract well-worn grooves of au-tomatic, unthinking behavior.

Still, in and of itself, awareness does not constitute change. It's possible to increase your awareness without changing your behavior. You may be fully conscious of the fact that you're going to stop at Dunkin' Donuts on the way to work or sit down with some cookie dough and a spoon at the end of a hard day, but you might not see how that knowledge can lead to change. We see a lot of clients who feel as though they get stuck on the way from awareness to new behavior. "I know exactly what I'm doing. Why on earth do I keep doing it?" asked one client during a mindful-eating group. The answer is usually multifaceted, and exploring the root causes (stress? negative body image? loneliness?) is an important part of the journey. But there's a more immediate question: *"How can I do something different?"*

We've talked a lot about how cultivating kind awareness opens up behaviors and realities you didn't realize were possible. One client, Jennifer, became aware that her habit of *occasionally* stopping for hot chocolate and a donut on the way home from work had become a *daily* habit. Her pattern changed when, one afternoon, she prepared a cup of spicy-sweet herbal tea for her commute home instead—a healthier choice that provided the comforting warmth and flavor without the calories and blood-sugar roller coaster. This change didn't "just happen," however. She arrived at this alternative after weeks of learning to recognize the multiple triggers—external and internal—that set up and reinforced the hot chocolate–donut pattern.

When you learn to truly pay attention to your environment as well as your body, your thoughts, and your emotions—without judgment and with kindness—you can find various points along the way where you can stop the spiral that leads to overeating. Whether or not you've experienced this expansion of perception and possibilities yet, you can learn how to do so, and how to follow through with choices that support your health rather than undermine it. This chapter provides the road map.

Understanding Your Triggers

Throughout *The Mindful Diet* you've been learning about the many factors that can lead to eating when we're not hungry, or eating past the point of fullness, and how those patterns get set in place through our behaviors, and then kept in place neurologically and environmentally. Everything from visual cues, to cooking smells, to social anxiety, to a need for stimulation can prompt us to eat.

Eating triggers are highly idiosyncratic. The situations that trigger overeating for one person may be irrelevant for another. For Patty, age 45, the smell of cookies baking is irresistible. "And I work next to a bakery!" she says. For Elizabeth, age 30, conversations with her volatile father propel her toward the kitchen, but she's not particular about *what* she eats; whatever's abundant will do—leftover lasagna, popcorn, crackers, or ice cream. For countless people, the McDonald's golden arches are a siren whose song seems to take control of their car's steering wheel, leading them into the drive-through for a dose of hot, salty, crunchy calorie bombs.

Through mindfulness practice and journaling exercises, you've been gathering data about your eating triggers. But there's knowing and there's *knowing*. The process we're going to take you through will help you to map out alternatives to the automatic habits that aren't serving you well; practicing these alternatives has the power to rewire your brain. Mindfulness meditation will support this rewiring. But first, you need to get really clear on your triggers.

Triggers come at us from both the outside world and our own thoughts, beliefs, and feelings. An overeating incident often encompasses a swirl of internal and external factors, and to get a handle on them, it's helpful to start by breaking them down. In the list below, you may recognize one or two main triggers, or you may identify with a dozen. People who have long-standing weight and eating issues tend to have multiple triggers. If this is the case for you, make an effort to avoid layering on judgment (*I have no willpower!*) or fear (*How will I ever get a handle on all those triggers?*). Instead, see the simple fact—that food has become a go-to "solution" for a whole host of situations, thoughts, and feelings.

External triggers

- Advertisements showing food or eating
- Baked goods, candy, and snacks in the workplace
- Working lunches or dinners
- "Problem" foods (e.g., chips or chocolate) that are readily available
- Certain times of day
- Friends or family eating
- Certain activities that have been paired with eating, such as watching TV or driving
- Certain people
- Family gatherings
- Others: _____
- _____
- _____

Internal triggers

- Childhood associations
- Chronic stress
- Anxiety
- Anger
- Hunger (especially when strong)
- Loneliness
- Negative feelings and thoughts about your body
- Harsh, self-critical thoughts
- All-or-nothing thinking
- Catastrophic beliefs
- Fatigue
- Boredom
- Pain
- Others: _____
- _____
- _____

Consider which of the above factors are eating triggers for you. It can help to look back through the food and feelings tracker in your journal and search for patterns. Does one theme emerge? Or are there several? Keep in mind that some of these triggers may be relatively immediate and discrete (such as phone calls with a difficult family member), whereas others may be more pervasive (such as loneliness).

Re-creating the Chain of Events

Having a sense of the external and internal factors that tend to trigger unhealthy eating can help you delve more deeply and see how your triggers interact. Mindfulness teaches change from the inside out, not the outside in—which means seeing and understanding what is happening in our bodies and minds. Using a technique called **chain analysis,** or **chaining,** we'll show you how to examine not only an unhealthy incident itself but, more important, the events, thoughts, and feelings that preceded it. When you do this, you'll find that typically an eating episode isn't an immediate reaction to a single trigger; it's a culmination of bundled reactions of sensations, thoughts, emotions, and behaviors.

Chain analysis teases apart the bundled reaction, yielding the "chain" of causes and effects that can culminate in a choice that's not in our best interest, such as overeating or skipping exercise. Consider Leya, age 32, who described bingeing on Thai food in front of the TV one night and then belittling herself afterward: "I turned on the TV and ate all the Thai food—every bite. It was blissfully distracting, until the last bite was gone and my stomach hurt. Then I felt horribly guilty and started berating myself for being so weak." She attributed the binge to her lack of willpower, but as you'll see below, when she worked backward to re-create the chain of events that led up to the incident, she discovered more than a dozen contributing factors—ranging from events (an argument with her husband) and behaviors (getting poor sleep and eating a minimal breakfast and lunch) to emotions (disappointment and sadness) to thoughts (criticizing her body).

The power of chain analysis lies in the fact that once you get good at recognizing the chain of events, *you can formulate alternatives*. Each link in the chain—be it an external stressor, a distorted thought, or an emotion—represents a "fork in the road," an opportunity to make a choice. And with enough practice, you can become aware of these choices not only in hindsight, but also in the moment. Eventually, you'll be able to see them coming.

Step 1: Constructing Your Chain

Many people find that working backward is the most useful approach to doing chain analysis, especially when you're learning it. You'll start with the overeating incident itself, then explore what happened right before *that*, and right before *that*, and so on. When we say "what happened," we mean not only external events but also internal "micro-events," such as thoughts and emotions—more on that below. This takes some time and thought—and a nonjudgmental, curious attitude. You'll notice that your skills at recognizing micro-events improve with your daily mindfulness practice. At first, when you think about an incident in which you ate too much or ate something unhealthy, you may perceive a confusing jumble of stressors, emotions, and temptations. Or it may seem like a simple lack of impulse control. But as you practice mindfulness, you will be training yourself to recognize the tiny pieces that make up what seems like a single event—the sensations, thoughts, feelings, and behaviors. So, even if you are aware of a major trigger, continued daily practice as well as this exercise will help to increase your awareness. Spend the time to work backward filling in the details, because you'll likely discover additional triggers—which ultimately mean additional opportunities to chart a new course.

When doing her chain analysis, Leya started with the overeating episode: *I binged on takeout Thai food while watching TV.*

Then she asked herself, "What happened just before that?" *Listened to voice mail; my husband left a message saying that he has to cover the night shift for a fellow resident. He says he's sorry. I'm flooded with disappoint-*

ment and frustration; I had wanted to resolve last night's argument. He's always working late.

And then, "What happened before that?" *I walked into our house, caught my reflection in the mirror and saw how gross my double chin looked. I felt disgusted with myself.*

And then, "What happened before that?" *I ran into an old friend with a newborn and felt overwhelming sadness about my own struggles getting pregnant; I felt annoyed with myself for feeling that way instead of just feeling happy for my friend.*

And then, "What happened before that?" *I completed the graphs I needed to design at work. Focused pretty well.*

And then, "What happened before that?" *I ate only a small side salad for lunch.*

And then, "What happened before that?" *I had meetings all morning, felt distracted and tired. Drank coffee all morning.*

And then, "What happened before that?" *Instead of taking my usual morning walk, which helps my stress levels, I thought "It's too cold" and skipped it.*

And then, "What happened before that?" *I didn't sleep well after arguing with my husband—and skipped breakfast.*

When doing chain analysis, it's the details that matter; each and every external situation, behavior, physical sensation, thought, and emotion is a "link" in the chain. In her journal, Leya broke down each basic event above into its components. Once she'd completed the process, she could see how the internal and external events fit together, and could ultimately reconstruct the series of "links" that led up to the overeating episode:

Argued with husband about money last night (behavior)
Felt sad (emotion)
Felt frustrated (emotion)
Slept poorly (behavior)
"It's too cold" (thought)
Skipped morning walk (behavior)

Skipped breakfast in order to get to work early (behavior)
Drank coffee throughout the morning (behavior)
Ate only a small salad for lunch (behavior)
Focused on work much of the afternoon (behavior)
Saw friend with baby (behavior)
Felt grief (emotion)
*"How ridiculous to feel sorry for myself instead of happy for my
    friend"* (thought)
Annoyed with self (emotion)
Exhausted at end of day (sensation)
Walked into house (behavior)
Looked in mirror and saw my chin (behavior)
"My double chin is gross" (thought)
Felt disgusted (emotion)
Listened to voice mail and got husband's message (behavior)
Felt disappointment (emotion)
"He always works late" (thought)
Felt frustration (emotion)
Felt disgusted (emotion)
Sat in front of TV to eat (behavior)
Ate all the Thai food straight from the container (behavior)

In reviewing the links, Leya could see a number of places that added to her vulnerability to eating all the Thai leftovers. We'll get there, but first it's your turn. In your journal, lay out the chain of links that preceded a recent eating event in which you ate more than you needed or made unhealthy choices—something within the last few days is ideal. If it's more distant than that, you will forget details, and effective chain analysis is all about the details. *It's the details that will help you discover the paths out.* Work backward to reconstruct the time that led up to the eating episode. Start by asking yourself, "What happened before that? . . . And before that?" to get the basics. Include events and behaviors (e.g., dinner with extended family, skipping exercise), thoughts (e.g., self-criticism about your body or your willpower, negative thoughts about something you did), feelings (e.g., anger, sadness), and physical sensations (e.g., tight neck, hunger, fullness, fatigue, pain).

Often, reconstructing the two days before the episode occurred is sufficient, but go as far back as you need to go. For example, if you overate at a brunch on Saturday after a very stressful week at work, include parts of the workweek if that seems relevant. Be as specific as you can. Did you have a difficult meeting? Did you "forget" to eat because you were so busy? Keep in mind things like inadequate sleep, other stressful situations, intense or chronic emotions, old habits, memories that disturb you, sensations you ignore, tempting food, et cetera. Be as specific as you can; use enough detail that an actor could re-create the scene.

It's useful to work in pencil because the more you explore, the more you'll fill in. Leave enough space between events and behaviors to add thoughts, emotions, and sensations.

Insights and Inspirations: Ellie, age 48

Chocolate is my weakness. Such a cliché, right? The problem is that I don't eat a piece of chocolate, I eat all the chocolate I can until it's gone. The last time I binged on chocolate was during a reunion with my college friends. When I arrived, I noticed our host had left a big jar of Hershey's kisses in everyone's room. After dinner, everyone was drinking, which I'd stopped doing ten years ago after going through breast cancer treatment. So everyone was laughing and telling old stories in that drunken way, and I ended up feeling very alone, not part of things. I went to bed early and saw the Hershey's kisses. Ten minutes later, the jar was empty. When I did chaining, though, I remembered having a very distinct thought when I arrived and saw the jar of chocolate: "Get this out of here"—and then talking myself out of doing anything. I didn't want to seem rude, and I didn't want to admit my vulnerability to these old friends, who were all thin and successful. I also realized that I went into the weekend with very little sleep, and fatigue is a big trigger for overeating for me. So it was really a culmination of things.

What Do You *Really* Need?

Reconstructing events through chain analysis puts into sharp relief the fact that *what we feel we need in the moment is often at odds with our true need.* What do we mean by this? That chocolate bar, that TV show, curling up on the couch—those things can all seem nurturing and comforting in the moment. But are they what we really need? When Leya responded to the chilly weather by forgoing her usual morning walk, she was responding to a short-term "need" . . . an immediate desire for comfort. But her true, long-standing need is stress relief—and her daily walk is an important part of meeting that need. Perhaps she could have worn a heavier coat. Thinking long-term is challenging in a fast-paced society, but *absolutely essential for self-care.*

There aren't hard-and-fast rules about needs; it's about context and knowing yourself. Think about the long-term consequences of your choices. **Is what you're doing addressing an immediate wish or need but undermining a bigger, longer-term need?** For example, imagine that you are planning to exercise, but feel so tired or down that it seems too hard to muster the energy. If, instead of exercising, you decide to drop onto the couch to "rest and just be comfortable," you are responding to your immediate need, but whether or not you are truly taking care of yourself depends on the context. Do you actually need more sleep? Or do you need more energy? Exercise can help with both energy and sleep quality. If you had only two hours of sleep the night before because you were up late working on a project, however, it may make more sense to take a nap than to exercise. But if you're succumbing to your default—your automatic pattern that you want to change—you're probably not addressing your true, long-term need by resting on the couch.

Recognizing and prioritizing your true needs requires checking in with your Inner Compass and listening for your "wise mind" so that, eventually, it speaks louder than your "I want it now," immediate-gratification-oriented lower brain. Neurologically, it's about circumventing the powerful limbic-system forces that drive so much behavior and have the potential to undermine our health. Energetically, it's about shifting the power to the part of us that wants to change.

In the chain analysis example, Leya's true need was a combination of companionship, comfort, and hunger. In the chain you built, what, in hindsight, do you believe your true need was? Think about the bigger context of your life. Also, write down strategies to meet this need in a healthier way in the future. Be honest with yourself, and you may be surprised at the amount of power that you possess to make a difference in what appear to be "automatic" and "out-of-control" behaviors.

Step 2: Mapping the Alternatives

Once you've identified the series of automatic reactions through chain analysis, you can identify alternatives at many points along the way. Because you're looking back at an event with kindness and curiosity, chaining allows for perspective that is not always there in the moment. Each link signifies a fork in the road at which you can either fall into old patterns or chart a new course. Alternatives can take many forms—from *actions,* such as taking a different route home so that you don't drive past Dunkin' Donuts, to *managing your thoughts,* such as identifying a self-critical thought as such (reminding yourself that it's just a thought that the mind creates) and questioning it rather than reacting to it. Other times, you're actively creating new options, such as bringing healthy snacks to work every day. A given alternative might seem inconsequential, but each time you do something different, you're shifting away from the well-worn path that leads to unhealthy eating behavior. Physiologically, you're starting to create new neural pathways.

For **external triggers** such as passing by your neighborhood ice-cream place, avoidance of the trigger can be an effective alternative, at least in the short term. Avoiding triggers isn't always possible or realistic—as in the case of Patty, who works next to a bakery. But even small changes in your patterns can have powerful effects. For example, Kristen, who always went straight to the fridge after work, realized during chaining that she could go into her house through the side door, bypassing the kitchen altogether. This small change helped her shift her pattern. Having healthy foods on hand is another common behavioral alternative for office-related triggers such as vending machines and baked goods. After you practice a new pattern for a while—laying down new neural pathways in your brain—an external trigger tends to lose some of its power, and you probably won't need to avoid it.

Internal triggers, such as thoughts and emotions, are more subtle but no less powerful. Let's start with thoughts. Like behavioral patterns, thought patterns have neural pathways. Your mindfulness practice makes you more aware of your thoughts, and how they're part of your eating patterns. When doing chaining, make an effort to recall your thoughts. (This is why picking a recent event is helpful.) While you may not be able to prevent a thought from occurring, you can remember that a thought is just a mental event—not truth. Our minds constantly chatter, and much of what they say is not truth. Just observing the chatter and recognizing a specific thought or judgment as "only a thought" can diminish its power. You can also question the thought ("Is this true?") or choose to just let it pass without giving it much attention.

Take Leya's thought about her chin—that it's "gross." Reminding herself that her mind just created that judgment, likely out of habit, and asking herself, "What's the data here and what is a story or judgment?" and "Is this thought helping me reach my goal?" are powerful alternatives to reacting to the thought as if it were true. By not engaging with or believing the old thought, and by asking yourself a new question ("What is true?"), you're taking a detour out of the old pathway that is not serving your health. Remember, self-critical judgments, which are pervasive in people struggling with weight and eating issues, counteract the momentum of change.

Emotions tend to sweep us quickly and powerfully into reactive behavior. But your mindfulness practice has given you the experience of "seeing" your emotions and finding a distance between feeling and act-ing. That distance is key to developing alternatives. When you're doing the chaining exercise and come across an emotion that you reacted to in an unhealthy way—such as anger, anxiety, or sadness—ask yourself, "What else could I have done in that moment to manage that emotion?" As with thoughts, simply relating to the emotion in a new way—having distance from it instead of being swept away by it—provides an important transition between automatic behavior and choices that move you toward your goals. Alternatives for emotional triggers include observing the emotion instead of reacting to it (you might notice that it rises and falls) and offering yourself kindness and compassion. You can also think about how you might address the true need the emotion signals. For example, when you're feeling lonely, you might need to reach out to a friend. When frustrated, a ten-minute meditation may help calm you down and allow you to find new perspectives. Physical exercise can help to dissolve the energy of emotion, especially if you take a mindful approach and shift your focus from the emotion to sensation—just feel your body moving through space.

When Leya reflected on the Thai food incident, she realized that she had fallen into an old pattern of not eating enough at breakfast and lunch—which set her up for overeating at night. She also realized that instead of feeling annoyed with herself for being sad about her fertility struggles, she needed to give herself some space and compassion for those feelings.

For all types of triggers—internal and external—returning to and remembering your values is essential for formulating alternatives that you'll actually act upon. For Leya, inner peace was one of her values; coming back to that could help her figure out strategies for talking to her husband about sensitive subjects and for setting herself up for less stressful workdays.

Go back to your exercise and add alternatives beside every link in the chain that you can. Write in a choice that could have altered the chain of events somewhere in the link. Draw from your mindfulness toolkit (see the chart below for ideas). Put in multiple alternatives when possible.

Breaking the Chain

Type of trigger	Example	Alternatives
External Triggers		
Surroundings	Walking past favorite restaurant Other people eating Presence of certain foods	Avoid the trigger; consciously distance yourself from it. Do a Mini-Meditation to stay clear on whether or not to eat. Do a Hunger-Fullness Scan. Eat only if hungry. Eat a small portion and stop. Focus on taste satiety. Have alternative foods available.
Internal Triggers		
Thoughts	Self-criticism Judgments about your body Thoughts/obsessions about certain foods All-or-nothing statements, such as "I have no willpower" or "I can't . . ."	Recognize the thought. Is it data or a story? Do a Body Scan to experience rather than judge the body. Ask yourself: Is this true? How do I know? Let the thought pass without engaging it.

		Ask yourself: Does it help me attain my goal? Use your Inner Compass.
Emotions	Sadness, fear, anger Feeling-thought combinations like anxiety and frustration Loneliness	Allow yourself to feel the emotion without doing anything or judging it; notice when it dissipates. Ask yourself, "What's my true need?" Address your true need: call a friend; exercise Do a Loving-Kindness Meditation. If you must eat, eat a small portion and stop. Focus on taste satiety.
Physical sensations	Fatigue Pain Hunger Low energy Tension	Do a Body Scan. Observe sensations without reacting to them. Do a Hunger-Fullness Scan. If hungry, eat until first sign of fullness. Address your true need: sleep; deep rest; eating (if hungry); treat pain if possible (medication, massage, acupuncture); exercise; stretch

When Leya looked back at her chain, she came up with a number of alternatives:

- *Instead of talking to my husband about money at night, I could have suggested tabling the discussion until the weekend when we had time and were less stressed. That might have helped me sleep more soundly and be less upset.*

- *After our argument, I could have done a short meditation or yoga instead of staring at the ceiling and stewing.*

- *When I thought, "It's too cold for a walk," I could have examined that thought and compared it with my true need (stress relief).*

- *When I thought to myself, "No time for breakfast," I could have asked, "Is that really true?" I could have made myself a simple breakfast— whole-wheat toast and almond butter—despite being rushed.*

- *Instead of coffee (which tends to amp up my stress), I could have had tea.*

- *At lunchtime, I could have ordered something more substantial than a salad. Doing a Hunger-Fullness Scan might have helped too.*

- *After running into the friend with the baby, I could have been com- passionate toward myself for being sad about my fertility struggles, instead of feeling annoyed with myself.*

- *When telling myself that my chin was "gross," I could have stepped back and recognized that I was having a judgmental thought—and that it was the voice of my Inner Critic.*

- *Upon listening to my husband's voice mail and feeling that tidal wave of emotion, I could have done any of a number of things (besides sit down with the Thai food)—taken a walk, paged him so that we could check in, meditated and let the emotions rise and fall, asked my neighbor over for company—or even all of these things.*

- *Instead of eating in front of the TV, I could have eaten in the kitchen or dining room.*

- *Instead of eating out of the takeout container, I could have served myself a small portion.*

- *Instead of eating quickly, I could have eaten slowly and really at- tended to every bite.*

- *I could have saved the Thai food for tomorrow, to share with my husband, and eaten a bowl of turkey chili left over from last night.*
- *Instead of berating myself for overeating, I could have observed what had happened and offered myself compassion, maybe doing a Loving-Kindness Meditation.*

Insights and Inspirations: Kara, age 41

I can't tell you how many times I've tried to eat less and exercise more. But it was always about imposing a plan, willing myself to "just do it." I was on the wagon, then off, then on, then off—for twenty years. This time it's about paying attention—to everything, really—and there's no wagon to fall off of. When I'm really paying attention, I can hear the voice that really does want to change, and knows why. I realize how many choices I actually have at any given moment. It feels like I'm awake for the first time.

Step 3: Putting It Together in the Moment

When combined with your mindfulness practice, doing chain analysis will help you understand and predict your patterns. Instead of having your reactions "sneak up on you" and unfold, you'll have anticipated them. After you've done the chaining exercise several times, you will see similar situations, reactions, thoughts, and feelings start to emerge. But this time, you'll have strategies for each trigger and reaction at the ready.

Leya saw that stress reactivity was the primary driver in her overeating episode and realized that was a common pattern for her. She upped her meditation practice from fifteen minutes to twenty-five minutes and found that this helped her manage her thoughts and emotions (specifically, frustration and disappointment). The next time she and her husband had a disagreement, she felt much calmer while they were talking; afterward, she did 20 Breaths, which helped her to relax enough to go to sleep. She also began to question one of her frequent thoughts, "I don't have time for breakfast," and saw that it diverged from her true need: energy and steady blood-sugar levels for a busy workday. She made time for eating breakfast, and to prepare for especially hectic days, she stocked her glove compartment and office drawer with baggies of raw nuts.

Insights and Inspirations: Lilian, age 62

I used to feel like my overeating episodes "just happened"—like I had no choice, almost like I was possessed. But now I know exactly what's happening when it's happening. And there are a dozen ways to do it differently. Befriending my feelings. Recognizing my thoughts. Just sitting at the table instead of in front of the TV to eat has been powerful for me. And I know that it actually is possible to eat one cookie and not twelve. There's a big difference between eating one cookie and eating twelve! I ask myself whether what's "good for me" right now is what's good for me in the long run.

You may come up against triggers that feel pervasive and overwhelming. For Holly, whose husband died five years ago, the main trigger was loneliness. When she felt very lonely, she would put on her pajamas and decide to withdraw from the world. This set her up for a big eating binge, which comforted her in the moment and then made her feel worse. Of course, she wasn't going to cure her loneliness with a single alternate choice. But when she was in touch with her wise mind, her values, and her true needs, she saw that the way to counteract the feeling of loneliness in the moment was to reach out—call a friend or even go to a bookstore or a café and be around strangers. These alternatives gave her genuine comfort in the moment—she was responding to her *true need* for human contact. And the energy and confidence she gained from shifting that pattern helped her start to build new relationships.

Know-Your-Triggers Cheat Sheet

- *Before* going into a situation that's likely to trigger you (a stressful meeting, a night alone, a cocktail party), think about the triggers and your usual reactions. Ask yourself, "How can I prepare for this situation?"
- When you *experience a trigger*, use your mindfulness skills to step back and see what is happening, and think about the alternatives you've mapped out. Do the 20 Breaths exercise to create some space and calm. If you still feel pulled toward your usual reaction, take a moment to check in with your values and goals. What action, thought, or feeling is going to help you reach your goals and live according to your values?

A New Structure, Inside and Out

Without sufficient support and structure in place, inside our minds and in our environments, we lapse into old patterns. This isn't character weakness; it's neurochemistry and environment. The human brain is not designed to run by willpower alone. To create new patterns, you need to build a new inner and outer infrastructure that supports those patterns.

Your mindfulness practice and skills—the ability to focus your attention on what is happening in the moment, bodily, emotionally, and mentally without judgment—represent the foundation of your new internal infrastructure. By practicing these skills, you begin to welcome emotions with kindness and meet thoughts with curiosity.

Clarifying your goals and values, and keeping them at the forefront of your thoughts, is another crucial building block, the beams and walls on top of the foundation. Mapping alternative choices through chaining—and then trying those choices—will help to solidify your new inner structure.

Your Mindfulness Toolkit

- 20 Breaths
- Mini-Meditation
- Daily Sitting Meditation
- Loving-Kindness Meditation
- Body Scan
- Hunger-Fullness Scan
- Taste Awareness
- Healing Self-Touch

In the next chapter, we'll delve more deeply into the external framework: what to eat to support a healthy weight and good overall health, and how to set up your environment and your life to support healthy habits. Each choice we make—savor a bite of dessert or eat the whole serving, cook or go out to dinner, make a meal or pop a frozen pizza in the oven—is a movement toward or away from what we want for our bodies, our health, and our lives.

PART III

Eating for Total Health

CHAPTER 10

The Four Pillars of Healthy Eating

"We are indeed much more than what we eat,
but what we eat can nevertheless help us to
become much more than what we are."

—Adelle Davis

Awareness and intention lie at the heart of lasting change. By now you've begun the process of recognizing your deeply ingrained eating patterns and building new ones. You've been learning to pay attention to why you eat and how you eat, to understand your internal and external triggers, and to listen to what's happening in your body and your mind. You've learned how to recognize the diet mentality and use the power of mindfulness to slow down your automatic behaviors and make different, healthier choices. And you've learned to connect the dots between what's happening in your life—your mood and stress levels in particular—and what and how much you end up eating. The skills and wisdom you've gained are your foundation for lasting change.

Now it's time to start building a way of eating that truly supports your health. That means, in addition to knowing *when* to eat, knowing *what* to eat. You might think it's obvious or that it will take care of itself—just eat the healthy stuff! But in today's world, eating a healthy diet takes knowledge, planning, and most important, intention. What has become the "default" diet in this country, the food that surrounds us and is easily accessed, gets people in serious trouble with their weight and their health.

Food is *powerful*. Research confirms that the impact of our diet on our health goes far beyond a simplistic "calories-in-versus-calories-out" equation or getting sufficient vitamins and minerals. In fact, your body is a biochemical environment that is deeply affected by what you eat and drink. Your body knows the difference between a handful of nuts and a candy bar, or between a homemade vegetable stir-fry and a frozen pizza. How? The compounds we take in—whether the antioxidants in blueberries or the preservatives in a Dorito—ultimately wash over our DNA and influence gene expression. A thousand calories of blueberries sends much different signals than a thousand calories of Doritos. Over time, what you eat and drink either supports or distorts the healthy functioning of your body. The chemistry is complicated, but what it boils down to is simple: **Everything you put in your body matters.**

Processed, fried, and high-sugar foods have become the status quo diet for adults, teenagers, and even children. This combination of unhealthy foods, known as the standard American diet (SAD), not only leads to weight gain but also sends the wrong signals to our DNA. Over time, this affects the proper functioning of all our body's systems. From a public-health perspective, the SAD is a disaster that's led to epidemic rates of obesity, prediabetes and diabetes, heart disease, and certain types of cancer. In short, our cultural diet plays a major role in the chronic, life-threatening conditions that affect about half of American adults—SAD indeed.

The good news is that the eating principles we teach have an equal and opposite effect on your body: they build your health and vitality from your cells on up and naturally guide you toward a healthy weight. Following those principles does not mean you have to eat perfectly all the time or that there's no place for convenience or indulgence. Rather, it means that the *majority* of what passes through your lips should be foods and beverages that support your health. The result? Your odds for excellent health *and* a healthy weight skyrocket.

The Status Quo Diet: How Did We Get Here?

Just a few hundred years ago, most people subsisted on vegetables and fruits, whole grains, legumes, fish, and sometimes meat. But as the agriculture and food industries began to expand to accommodate a changing, more mobile society, a glut of far less wholesome foods started to work their way into the American diet. Manufacturers found that if they removed certain parts of foods and added other ingredients, such as preservatives, foods could be shipped greater distances with less spoilage.

As our culture shifted and processed food became widely available, our taste preferences shifted. We got turned on to refined sugar, refined oils, and refined grains as corner markets morphed into supermarkets, then into big-box stores. Meat emerged as a mainstay, and industrial farms began feeding their animals more cost-efficient grains instead of their traditional grasses and adding growth hormones to boost production and profits. Fast food became a cultural staple, as did processed foods devoid of nutrients but crammed with salt, sugar, and synthetic chemicals.

Today, most of the calories Americans consume each day come from refined grains, added sugars, vegetable oils, and solid fats—much of it in the form of foods that did not exist one hundred years ago. Consider sugar: whereas our ancestors ate very little refined sugar—about twenty teaspoons a year by some estimates—today Americans consume on average more than twenty-two teaspoons *a day*, much of it in the form of a highly processed variety called high-fructose corn syrup. Besides the calorie burden and the harmful effects of these foods, they're taking the place of foods that are essential to the proper functioning of our bodies— nutrient-rich foods like fruits and vegetables, which help us age well and reduce our risk of disease. Less than 25 percent of adults report eating five or more servings of fruits and vegetables per day.

America's Top 10

According to the USDA, the leading sources of calories for adults in the United States are as follows:

- Grain-based desserts
- Breads
- Chicken and chicken dishes
- Sodas and energy beverages
- Alcoholic beverages
- Pizza
- Tortillas, burritos, and tacos
- Pasta and pasta dishes
- Beef and beef dishes
- Dairy desserts

Our guidelines are based on inclusion—meaning that instead of focusing on what *not* to eat, we focus on the foods that our bodies were designed to eat—foods that will naturally promote a healthy weight and good overall health. While we all have genetic "blueprints" that we inherit and are all a bit different in terms of what influences our choices, the science tells us that **a healthy diet is built on four key attributes: it's anti-inflammatory, it leads to balanced blood sugar, it's made up of whole foods, and it's plant-based.** Here, we'll explain what eating based on these four pillars does for your body on a biochemical level and why following them is easier than you think.

Pillar 1: Eat to Manage Inflammation

If you follow health news, you've heard about the links between inflammation and illness. Recent research has found a certain type of inflammation—chronic, low-grade, and systemic—to be an underlying cause of many conditions that are epidemic in this country. Heart disease, certain cancers, type 2 diabetes, Alzheimer's disease, and obesity are among the conditions that have been linked to chronic inflammation. In and of itself, however, inflammation is not the problem; in fact, human beings would not have survived the last 2.5 million years without this complex and life-saving response.

Say you burn your hand taking a pan out of the oven, injure your shoulder, or catch a virus. The redness, heat, swelling, or fever you feel is **acute inflammation**—the cornerstone of the body's immune system. As part of a highly organized healing response, **inflammatory compounds** increase swelling, aid in blood clotting, constrict blood vessels, and catalyze processes to fight infection (in the case of a virus) or repair damaged cells (in the case of a burn or injury). When our bodies are functioning normally, the inflammation subsides when the injury or illness is resolved. At that point, the immune system releases **anti-inflammatory compounds,** which reduce swelling, relax blood vessels, and improve blood flow.

When our bodies are *not* functioning normally, the immune system sometimes churns out inflammatory compounds *even when there's no infection to fight off or overt injury to heal*—for years or even decades. This condition, known as **chronic inflammation,** is the body's response to cell damage that occurs from a wide array of triggers—including UV radiation, environmental toxins, and certain foods at the heart of the SAD (in particular, refined carbohydrates, sugars, and unhealthy fats). Insufficient sleep, sedentary lifestyles, and chronic stress—what has unfortunately become the "standard American lifestyle"—also contribute to chronic inflammation.

Whereas acute inflammation is localized within the body, chronic inflammation affects *the entire body*. Inflammatory compounds rove through your system 24/7, seeking to repair the damage caused by the triggers above. These compounds inadvertently harm healthy tissue, including blood vessels and organs, and even our DNA, increasing the risk of heart disease, cancer, diabetes, Alzheimer's, and autoimmune diseases.

Chronic inflammation is intertwined with excess weight and obesity in a kind of vicious cycle. Not only can inflammation make it harder to lose weight, but a growing body of research reveals that simply carrying too much extra fat can increase inflammation. As fat accumulates, particularly in and around the abdomen, a class of immune cells called macrophages enter fatty tissue and prompt the release of inflammatory compounds. Abdominal fat is essentially its own source of chronic, low-grade inflammation.

We cannot control all of the myriad triggers for chronic inflammation. Therefore, we need to look at the factors we *can* control. We can limit our exposure to toxins and pollutants, use sunscreen (to protect from UV damage), and commit to daily practices that help us to relax and get restorative sleep. (Revisit chapter 7 if you need a refresher.)

What we eat and drink plays a major role in either cooling or fueling the fires of the inflammatory process. By minimizing the foods and preparation methods that trigger inflammation and maximizing your intake of foods that protect your cells from inflammation's damaging effects, you'll have an easier time losing weight and keeping it off, as well as protecting against inflammation-related diseases. There's even evidence that keeping inflammation in check may benefit your mood.

Quiz: How Inflammatory Is Your Diet?

The following eating habits may increase your risk for chronic inflammation. Check all that apply. (See page 294 for serving sizes.)

I rarely eat whole foods; most come from a package. ❑

I drink sodas or artificially sweetened beverages daily. ❑

I regularly use vegetable, corn, or soy oil in cooking. ❑

I consume baked goods, candy, or other sweets daily. ❑

I eat fewer than five servings of vegetables per day. ❑

I eat fewer than two servings of fruit per day. ❑

I do not eat green leafy vegetables or cruciferous
    vegetables four or more times a week. ❑

I eat grilled meat more than twice a week. ❑

I rarely/never eat cold-water fish (such as wild salmon,
cod, and sardines). ❑

I eat nuts, seeds, and avocado less than three times a week. ❑

If you checked any of the above, consider how you can shift to an anti-inflammatory diet instead. Use the strategies discussed in this section, and stay tuned for more ideas throughout this section of the book.

Choose Healthy Fats

As we discussed in chapter 3, dietary fat was demonized in a misguided nutrition campaign in the 1970s and 1980s. In fact, dietary fats are important for the proper functioning of our bodies. Our brains, the structure of every cell in the body, our metabolism, and our production of vitamins, neurotransmitters, and hormones depend on fats. **Essential fats** are those that must be provided in the diet, while nonessential fats, though important, can be made from other fats we consume.

Fats also provide the building blocks for our immune system. The type of fat you eat determines the degree to which your body will produce inflammatory or anti-inflammatory compounds—either stoking your body's inflammation or cooling it down. The family of fats referred to as **omega-6 fatty acids** are essential fats that provide support (building blocks) for the inflammatory compounds, while **omega-3 fatty acids** (also essential fats) support the formation of anti-inflammatory compounds.

Whereas our ancestors' diets naturally provided a balance of fats, the SAD has tipped the scales toward inflammatory fats. Roam the center aisles of your grocery store and you'll find scores of packaged foods made with refined vegetable oils like corn, cottonseed, safflower, and soybean oil. Each of these oils is high in omega-6 fatty acids. Animal products, from meats to cheese, also contain high levels of omega-6s called arachidonic acid (even more so when the animals are fed a grain-based diet). While omega-6s are vital to health—they support the body's *acute* inflammatory response—overdoing them can contribute to *chronic* inflammation. Trans fats, man-made fats found in many processed foods and fried foods—anything containing partially hydrogenated oil—also stoke inflammation. (See "Unwholesome Ingredients" on page 222 for more on trans fats.)

Fortunately, omega-3 fatty acids help quash the production of pro-inflammatory compounds. These good-for-you fats, the foundation of an anti-inflammatory diet, are abundant in oily fish (such as wild salmon, trout, herring, mackerel, and sardines) and plant foods like flaxseed, chia seeds, pumpkin seeds, hemp seeds, and walnuts.

Scientists theorize that our ancestors thrived on a diet with a 1:1 to 2:1 ratio of omega-6s to omega-3s. Thanks largely to an increased affection for the vegetable-oil-saturated processed foods described above—and to a drop-off in consumption of omega-3-rich fish—that ratio eventually skewed to 15:1 for the average American (and upward of 20:1 for those whose diets are based largely on processed refined foods). Rather than ruling out omega-6 fatty acids altogether, we emphasize scaling back on them while bumping up your intake of omega-3s. Research shows that the greater your body's supply of omega-3s is, the fewer omega-6s end up getting converted to inflammatory compounds.

Eat More Plants

Like omega-3s, plant foods nourish your body with naturally occurring anti-inflammatory compounds. Eating vegetables, fruits, grains, legumes and beans, and herbs and spices with a wide variety of colors, flavors, and aromas provides an abundance of plant compounds that have both anti-inflammatory and antioxidant benefits in your body. (We'll describe the amazing benefits of plant foods in greater depth later in this chapter.)

Omega-6 fats	Animal Sources	Plant Sources
Promote inflammation Constrict blood vessels Increase swelling and pain Induce fever Reduce circulation	Conventional eggs Conventional meat Poultry Dairy	Cottonseed Soybeans Palm Corn Grapeseed Sunflower seed (All used in refined vegetable oils; check labels on packaged foods.)

Omega-3 fats	Animal Sources	Plant Sources
Promote anti-inflammatory response Improve circulation Relax blood vessels Decrease muscle spasms and sensitivity to pain Reduce blood stickiness and blood clotting	Wild salmon Black cod Sardines Mackerel Anchovies Herring Meat and dairy products from grass-fed animals Omega-3-fortified eggs	Flaxseed (ground) Chia seeds Hemp seeds Algae Green leafy vegetables Pumpkin seeds Walnuts

Reduce Unhealthy Carbohydrates

Along with amping up your intake of anti-inflammatory fats and plants, it's essential to phase out refined carbs, sweets, and artificially or sugar-sweetened beverages—all of which increase inflammation. You'll benefit from cutting down on sugar (both in obvious sources and packaged foods that contain sugar) and choosing whole grains instead of the refined variety you find in white bread, white rice, and white pasta. Also make an effort to cut down on all flour-based products (like bread and pasta) in favor of **intact grains**—those that have not been ground into flour—such as brown rice, quinoa, and barley. While whole-grain breads and pastas are better for you than their refined counterparts, intact grains are better for your blood sugar and create less inflammation than flour-based products.

Consider Your Cooking Methods

How you cook counts, too. When meats are cooked at particularly high temperatures (by broiling, frying, or grilling, for instance), inflammatory compounds known as advanced glycation end products (AGEs) may be created. Linked to diabetes and hardening of the arteries in recent studies, AGEs appear to form at significantly lower levels when you simmer, poach, stew, or slow-cook your meat.

Pillar 2: Eat for Blood-Sugar Balance

Like chronic inflammation, a condition known as insulin resistance is increasingly common among Americans and closely linked to obesity and chronic illness. As with inflammation, what you eat can either help stabilize your blood-sugar levels or, over time, set you up for insulin resistance and its many attendant health troubles, including prediabetes and diabetes, metabolic syndrome, and heart disease.

Insulin, a hormone produced by the pancreas, is the key that unlocks your cells and allows them to absorb glucose, the sugar that serves as your body's main energy source. The carbohydrates you eat are broken down during digestion into smaller units—glucose, fructose, and galactose—which then enter your bloodstream and head to the liver. The liver then converts them all to glucose, which is either stored in the liver as glycogen or released into the bloodstream as needed throughout the body. When your pancreas detects this blood-sugar increase, it releases insulin, which helps to move glucose from your blood to the interior of your cells, where it's needed for energy. But in some people, a condition called insulin resistance develops, in which the body's cells become less responsive to insulin and the normal amount of insulin secreted is not sufficient to facilitate the movement of glucose into your cells. Hence, blood-sugar levels continue to rise, and because your pancreas keeps detecting high levels of glucose in your blood, insulin levels soar as well.

This is a very unhealthy situation for your body. Your cells are being robbed of the fuel they need to function properly; they are essentially starving. Because your cells can't get the right amount of glucose (aka sugar) into them, they may signal that they *need* sugar; one of the telltale signs of insulin resistance is a fierce craving for carbohydrates. Weight gain often results for a number of reasons: you may naturally reach for easily digested carbs to bring your energy level back up (compounding the problem); your cells begin slowing your metabolism in order to accommodate the decrease in energy supply; and, because insulin is a storage hormone, it causes your body to store extra glucose as fat (theoretically for later use). Most—but not all—people with insulin resistance are overweight or obese, according to a recent report from the Stanford University School of Medicine, and cardiovascular risk factors are significantly greater in people who are both overweight/obese and insulin-resistant.

When left unchecked, insulin resistance can lead to several chronic illnesses. First, the high blood-sugar levels set the stage for prediabetes and diabetes. Second, insulin resistance promotes the development of heart disease. In addition, since insulin influences the functioning of other hormones (such as estrogen and progesterone), it may be a key factor in certain hormone-related health problems (such as polycystic ovarian syndrome, a condition estimated to affect up to 5 million American women). What's more, insulin resistance puts major stress on your pancreas; researchers have been investigating a link between insulin resistance and pancreatic cancer.

Often, there are physical signs of insulin resistance, such as dark patches of skin on the front and back of the neck, elbows, knees, and knuckles. For some people, however, the signs are more subtle. Fatigue and a feeling of anxiety or jitteriness are common. If you suspect that you may be insulin resistant and/or have family members who are pre-diabetic or diabetic, talk to your health care provider about it. While certain genes may predispose you to insulin resistance, a diet packed with the wrong kind of carbs can also, over time, increase your risk. Since refined, non-nutritious carbs are a hallmark of the standard American diet, we're *all* vulnerable to insulin resistance. We emphasize carefully choosing carbs to give you energy while fending off insulin resistance—and helping you find your way to a healthy weight.

Quiz: Are You at Risk of Developing Insulin Resistance?

In our food environment, we're all potentially at risk of developing insulin resistance, and the factors below can contribute. If you're concerned about insulin resistance, talk to your doctor about whether diagnostic tests are warranted. Check all of the statements below that apply to you.

Most of the grains I eat are refined. ❑

I eat a lot of bread (more than four pieces per day). ❑

I eat sweets every day. ❑

I drink one or more diet or regular sodas a day. ❑

I often eat carbohydrate-only meals or snacks (pasta, crackers, pretzels, cheese puffs). ❑

I don't get regular aerobic exercise (exercise that gets the heart working, such as brisk walking, jogging, rowing, cycling, or swimming). ❑

I crave carbohydrates, often in the late afternoon. ❑

I often feel sleepy after meals, particularly those that contain
    more carbohydrates (breads, rice, pasta, fruits). ❑

I have a family history of diabetes. ❑

I tend to carry extra weight around my abdomen. ❑

I feel fatigued quite often. ❑

I have difficulty losing weight. ❑

I have high blood pressure. ❑

I have high triglycerides. ❑

I feel as if I have "brain fog." ❑

I have been told that my blood-sugar levels are "borderline." ❑

If you checked two or more boxes, follow up with your health care provider to discuss your risk factors.

Eating for Blood-Sugar Balance

The key to preventing (or reversing) insulin resistance and keeping your blood sugar under control is limiting your carbohydrate intake to foods that won't cause a quick spike in blood-sugar or insulin levels. For the most part, this means getting your carbs in the form of whole foods that contain plenty of fiber, such as vegetables, intact grains, beans, legumes, nuts, and seeds. With these foods, your body has to work to access the nutrients, digesting through fibrous outer layers, and glucose is released slowly and steadily. When you eat quickly digested carbs (refined grains, sugar-laden sweets, and super-starchy foods such as potatoes), however, your blood sugar spikes rapidly.

A tool called the **glycemic index** (GI) quantifies these differences. The GI is a ranking of carbohydrate-containing foods that indicates the degree to which they increase blood-sugar levels compared with drinking pure glucose. The scale goes from 1 to 100, and the higher the number, the more closely the food acts like pure sugar in your body. Whereas white rice (a refined grain) has a high glycemic index of 89, the GI of brown rice (an intact grain) is 50. White rice makes blood sugar spike; brown rice results in a more gradual rise in blood sugar. Beans, legumes, nonstarchy vegetables, and many fruits have a relatively low GI. **Glycemic load** (GL) uses the same principle but is more useful in that it takes into account the amount of food you're likely to eat; when applied to a meal, GL also includes the effect of other foods that accompany the meal—including proteins, fats, and fiber. For example, while carrots have a high GI when eaten alone, they are not generally consumed by themselves in great quantity, so their GL is moderate.

While GI and GL are useful tools, there's a simple, practical way to ensure that you're eating for optimal blood-sugar balance and overall health. **Every time you eat, aim for a combination of slow-burning carbohydrates (from vegetables, whole grains, and/or fruits), lean protein, and healthy fat.** That "magic formula" holds true for both meals and snacks. Instead of a big plate of pasta and a side of vegetables (mostly carbs), have a small amount of whole-grain or legume pasta with broccoli (carbs) and fish or chicken (protein), tossing in some pesto or avocado (healthy fat). Instead of grabbing just an apple (carbs) as a snack, have an apple with some almond butter (protein and fat).

Low-Glycemic Foods Work for Weight Loss

There's some evidence that eating predominantly low-glycemic foods might be your best bet for maintaining weight loss. In a study published in the *New England Journal of Medicine*, for instance, a high-protein, low-glycemic-load diet proved to be most effective in helping participants to maintain a healthy weight. A total of 772 families took part in the study, including 938 adults and 827 children. To set the stage for weight-loss maintenance, all overweight adults in the study followed a low-calorie diet for eight weeks, losing an average of about 24 pounds. Then, researchers placed all study members on one of five meal plans: a low-protein diet with a high GL, a low-protein diet with a low GL, a high-protein diet with a low GL, a high-protein diet with a high GL, or a control diet that involved no special instructions regarding GL levels. Results revealed that the high-protein, low-GL diet was superior to all other meal plans in keeping participants from gaining back the weight they'd shed in the first phase of the study. And this does not mean you need to exclude vegetables and fruits, as most of them have a low or moderate glycemic load—and they're essential for good health.

Move More

Eating well is essential for getting your blood sugar under control and decreasing your risk of developing insulin resistance, but so, too, is physical activity. There are so many reasons to move throughout the day: it lifts your mood, strengthens your bones, and improves your immune response. Exercise also changes the metabolism of your entire body. The more your body moves, the more glucose all of your muscles require. To meet this increased need, muscles are able to shuttle more glucose into their cells without having to rely only on insulin.

If you aren't exercising regularly yet, decide what you can realistically do this week. You might start with only ten minutes or twenty minutes a day. And it may help to think of it as *movement* as opposed to exercise at the start. Simply try to move your body more. Start with what you know you can accomplish and gradually build up to thirty to sixty minutes most days of the week. For most people, walking is the easiest thing to fit in, but dancing, swimming, and biking are also wonderful activities to work into your schedule. Many studies suggest that a combination of cardio exercise and strength training may be especially helpful in increasing insulin's efficiency and reversing insulin resistance.

Pillar 3: Eating Whole

The human body evolved to eat *food*—not refined food or man-made combinations of ingredients. In its whole natural state, brown or black rice can be a nutritional powerhouse. Whole rice is rich in fiber and delivers a host of B vitamins to support your heart, muscles, and digestive system. But like so many other grains, rice is often subject to a milling process to increase its shelf life, which does away with its bran and germ and all the precious nutrients held within. This "refined" rice is nutritionally bankrupt.

It's important to note that there's a wide spectrum of processed foods, ranging from minimally processed foods such as steel-cut oats to heavily processed foods such as frozen pizzas (see "Processed Foods: From Fortified to Frankenfoods," page 227). Whole foods contain a wealth of nutrients and phytochemicals (beneficial compounds in plants) that can sustain health and stave off sickness. And it's not just about what processing takes away from whole foods—it's also what gets added (salt, sugar, and synthetic chemicals) that's harmful to health (see "Unwholesome Ingredients," below).

What's more, thanks to clinical trials testing the use of supplements that contain isolated vitamins or minerals, we've learned that **synergy** may play a key role in the health-boosting benefits of certain foods. In other words, the good-for-you power of snacking on a handful of almonds might be due to its unique combination of vitamin E, magnesium, zinc, fiber, protein, and components that scientists don't yet understand. **Whole foods contain a delicate, inimitable interplay of nutrients and compounds that is absent in processed foods, even those fortified with added nutrients.**

Unwholesome Ingredients

While the crunch, sweetness, and shine of an apple may vary depending on the time of year or how far the fruit has traveled before landing in your palm, processed food is designed to deliver the same texture and taste in every bite—no matter how long it has lingered on the store shelf. It's worth taking a close look at what's responsible for the uncanny consistency of highly processed foods. Be mindful of ingredient lists and look out for these culprits:

Sodium. About 75 percent of the salt Americans consume each day comes from processed foods. Added to foods to draw out flavor, delay the growth of bacteria and mold, and mask the unsavory aftertaste of synthetic chemicals, all that sodium can raise your risk of cardiovascular disease and certain types of cancer (including stomach cancer). Taking in too much sodium can also prompt your body to leach calcium from your bones, leaving you more vulnerable to age-related bone thinning and osteoporosis.

Trans fats. In the early twentieth century, food manufacturers began adding hydrogen to vegetable oil to increase the time it took for the oil to turn rancid. Those hydrogenated oils, known as trans fats, have been shown to be more harmful to your heart than saturated fats. Responsible for the moist, gooey texture of packaged muffins, cookies, and cakes—and the crispness of foods such as potato chips, crackers, ramen noodles, and frozen foods—trans fats jack up your levels of LDL ("bad") cholesterol while driving down your levels of HDL ("good") cholesterol. Trans fats have also been shown to promote inflammation in the body within minutes of being consumed, raising and sustaining levels of the inflammation marker C-reactive protein hours after the meal, and setting the stage for the development of insulin resistance and diabetes. Recognizing these risks, the FDA has begun the process of removing trans fats from the food supply, but keep an eye out for "partially hydrogenated oil" on ingredient lists.

High-fructose corn syrup (HFCS). While we eat far too much sugar in all forms, high-fructose corn syrup is particularly unhealthy. HFCS is sweeter than regular corn syrup, thanks to processing methods that transform glucose to fructose (a super-sweet simple sugar not found in corn syrup in its natural form). Like trans fats, HFCS is cheap to make and highly favored by food manufacturers. It's abundant in sweet as well as savory foods, from sodas, ice cream, and jams to spaghetti sauce, lunch meats, and bread.

HFCS first hit American grocery-store shelves in the 1970s and is often linked to the start of the obesity epidemic in the United States. The body handles the digestion and absorption of HFCS differently than it does natural sources of fructose and glucose, and research suggests that consuming HFCS may contribute to a number of metabolic disturbances. Routine intake has been shown to promote the accumulation of body fat (especially around your belly). Moreover, unlike glucose, high-fructose corn syrup is metabolized by the liver, where it triggers the formation of triglycerides and cholesterol. Some of these lipids are stored, which can contribute to fatty liver disease; others are released into the bloodstream, elevating serum levels and increasing your risk of heart disease and other illnesses. There's also some evidence that HFCS might deplete your body's supply of chromium (a mineral involved in keeping levels of cholesterol, insulin, and blood sugar in check).

Synthetic chemicals. Eating whole means eating clean. Along with preservatives, dyes, and artificial flavoring and coloring agents, many processed foods contain synthetic sweeteners such as aspartame. Research shows that aspartame, for example, may threaten your nervous system by interfering with the normal signaling that occurs between nerve cells. A similar response has been noted with monosodium glutamate (MSG), another synthetic chemical commonly used as a food additive.

There are even some synthetic chemicals used in food *packaging* that could compromise your health. For instance, the tin used for some canned soups, fruits, and vegetables is often lined with bisphenol A (BPA), a toxin also used in the production of plastic water bottles. Mounting evidence shows that exposure to BPA (which appears to disrupt hormone function) could promote insulin resistance and the body-fat buildup emblematic of obesity.

The Fiber Factor

Fiber—the parts of plant foods that your body doesn't digest or absorb—is essential for optimal health. Fiber fosters heart health by lowering your levels of LDL ("bad") cholesterol, and possibly by reducing your blood pressure. A high fiber intake has also been found to be linked to low levels of C-reactive protein, an inflammation indicator, which suggests that fiber may help reduce inflammation in the body. Found to curb type 2 diabetes risk, a high-fiber diet is essential as well for slowing down your body's absorption of sugar and thus keeping glucose levels under control. Some studies even show that getting your fill of fiber may help thwart the development of colon cancer.

Two types of fiber are found in whole foods, soluble and insoluble. We need both to stay healthy, and most whole foods contain a mix. **Soluble fiber,** as its name implies, is soluble in water and forms a gel that helps to slow down digestion, delaying stomach emptying. This helps you to feel more full longer after eating and has a stabilizing effect on blood sugar, helping to improve insulin sensitivity. The gel-like property also acts to interfere with the absorption of dietary cholesterol.

Soluble fiber also contributes to a healthy population of beneficial bacteria in the gut, known as probiotics. It is estimated that the human body—the gastrointestinal tract in particular—is home to between five hundred and one thousand different species of these microbes. Recent studies have linked the makeup of our gut bacteria to weight, immune health, inflammation, chronic illness, and even mood. While much remains unknown about this emerging field of science, we do know that the soluble fiber that we consume through whole plants helps to support a healthy population of gut bacteria. When soluble fiber reaches the large intestine relatively undigested, it ferments, providing food for the probiotics and stimulating the growth of more beneficial bacteria. Soluble fiber is found in abundance in foods such as grains (barley, oats, oatmeal, or oat bran), legumes (dried beans, peas, or lentils), nuts, flaxseed, psyllium, fruits (apples, oranges, pears, or blueberries), and vegetables (cucumbers, carrots, or celery). Including probiotic-containing or fermented foods such as yogurt with active cultures, kefir, traditionally made sauerkraut, miso, and tempeh will further support a healthy balance of bacteria in your body.

Insoluble fiber, often referred to as "roughage," is not soluble in water. It tends to have a laxative effect while adding bulk to the diet, helping to speed gut transit and prevent constipation. For insoluble fiber, look to whole grains (such as brown rice and barley), wheat and corn bran, seeds and nuts, broccoli, cabbage, edible skins of fruits and vegetables, and dark green vegetables. Note that many fruits, vegetables, and whole grains contain both types of fiber.

Because eating fiber-rich foods tends to help you feel full, high-fiber diets are often closely linked to success in weight loss. You can experiment with fiber's effects on fullness for yourself in the exercise below.

Exercise: Fiber and Fullness Experiment

1. Using the Hunger-Fullness Scale, do this experiment: Drink 4 ounces of apple juice when you are moderately hungry (2.5 on the scale). Rate your hunger or fullness immediately afterward and record it in your journal.

2. The next day, eat one medium apple when you're moderately hungry and rate your hunger or fullness immediately afterward.

3. How did the two compare? Does the fact that the 4 ounces of juice and one medium apple are equivalent in calories surprise you?

The apple, a whole food, should have been more filling than the juice—and kept you full longer. The apple contains fiber, which fills you up, slows down your body's digestion, and leads to a relatively slow rise in blood sugar. Because apple juice contains no fiber, it isn't filling—and your body digests and absorbs it quickly, resulting in a rapid rise in blood sugar, followed by a rapid drop.

While "fiber-enriched" processed foods (including snack bars, cereals, and cookies) have gained in popularity in recent years—especially among dieters—research shows that such foods may do little to tame your hunger. In a recent study published in the *Journal of the Academy of Nutrition and Dietetics*, for instance, scientists found that fiber-fortified chocolate bars failed to increase satiety (but did cause uncomfortable side effects like gas and bloating in study participants). Again, isolating ingredients does not provide the benefits of whole foods. Rather than scouring labels, you can keep in mind Michael Pollan's advice: "Don't eat anything your great-grandmother wouldn't recognize as food."

Processed Foods: From Fortified to Frankenfoods

We're often asked, "Is everything that comes in a package bad?" The answer is no. Any food that has been handled or manipulated is a processed food. Bagged spinach, milk, fortified orange juice, and pre-chopped vegetables are all processed. But there's an enormous difference between these foods and heavily manipulated combinations of ingredients, such as frozen dinners.

Processed foods exist on a spectrum. On one end are whole foods that have been prepped for us, such as roasted nuts. These **minimally processed** foods can be an enormous time-saver and have a place in a healthy diet. On the other end are **heavily processed foods,** which we sometimes call Frankenfoods. These foods resemble nothing in nature and often contain dozens of ingredients used to thicken, color, preserve, stabilize, homogenize, or flavor the "food." They are also typically very high in added sodium, unhealthy fats, and sugar. In the middle are **moderately processed foods,** such as nut butter and dried fruit.

See the chart below for examples, but also keep in mind that with many foods, there's a spectrum of choices. Take bread. Many grocery stores sell freshly made bread that contains few ingredients—this would be moderately processed food. Wonder Bread, on the other hand, is heavily processed. Always read labels when you're buying packaged foods, and don't assume that labels such as "natural," "organic," or "vegetarian" mean that a food is healthy. Because the FDA doesn't define the term "natural," manufacturers can use it even when their products contain heavily processed ingredients. Packaged products that tout "organic ingredients" often also contain unhealthy oils or other man-made ingredients. One popular brand of vegetarian imitation-chicken nuggets contains *more than fifty* ingredients, including preservatives, stabilizers, and flavor enhancers: Frankenfood!

Minimally processed	Moderately processed	Heavily processed
Fresh, cut-up fruit	Fruit juice or dried whole fruit	Flavored fruit rolls or gummies
Pre-chopped vegetables	Fresh frozen vegetables	Frozen vegetable sides in sauces Veggie chips
Sardines	Salmon burgers	Fish sticks
Steel-cut oats	Instant oats	Toasted oat cereal
Shelled nuts	Nut butter	Peanut butter cup

Exercise: Track Your Processed Food Intake

1. Without trying to change your behavior, spend a week paying attention to how much of your diet is whole and how much is moderately or heavily processed. Write down everything you eat for breakfast, lunch, dinner, and snacks. And don't forget to keep using your hunger-fullness ratings as you do this. At the end of the week, make a list of all your whole foods

and all your packaged/processed foods. Which did you eat more of? What was the relationship between your fullness scores and whether you ate whole or processed foods?

2. Try to find two or three ways to shift toward whole foods. If you eat packaged breakfast cereal, for instance, try steel-cut oats with walnuts and blueberries. If you eat chips for an afternoon snack, try sugar snap peas with hummus. Instead of a frozen dinner, make a simple meal of roasted vegetables and fish or chicken.

Pillar 4: Eat a Plant-Based Diet

For much of history, human beings relied on the medicinal properties of plants to treat common maladies and maintain good health. Teeming with vitamins, minerals, and phytochemicals—natural compounds that protect and nourish your cells—plants are the foundation of a healthy diet. Today, more than ever, we need to eat "defensively"; a plant-based diet is our best weapon in helping our body cope with the effects of ongoing stress, inflammation, and exposure to environmental toxins. Studies show plant foods offer compounds that *change the expression of certain genes,* potentially stopping disease before it gets a foothold. By making plant foods the bedrock of your diet, you'll help to protect your body against illness and encourage a healthy weight.

Studies released in the last decade have shown us just how powerfully a plant-based diet contributes to good health. For a report published in the *American Journal of Clinical Nutrition,* for instance, Harvard School of Public Health researchers sized up the available studies on plant-based foods and prevention of cardiovascular disease. Their findings revealed that a high intake of plant-based foods is linked to significantly lower risk of coronary artery disease and stroke, and that following a plant-based diet featuring healthy fats, whole grains, omega-3 fatty acids, and a bounty of fruits and vegetables could be integral to preventing chronic disease. There's evidence that sticking to plant-based foods is key to easing inflammation; as noted earlier, vegetables and fruits have an anti-inflammatory effect, as do herbs and spices such as garlic, cinnamon, ginger, and turmeric. Eating plant foods also controls your blood sugar and protects against insulin resistance, reducing your diabetes risk. And some research, including one study from the *American Journal of Medicine*, suggests that following a plant-based diet could help promote weight loss, even without restrictions on portion size and calorie intake.

Plant foods—vegetables and fruits, whole grains, nuts, seeds, beans, legumes, herbs, and spices—serve as our most reliable source of the nutrients we need for overall health. And that includes protein, a macronutrient essential for building muscles and generating new cells, hormones, and antibodies. In the standard American diet, protein typically comes in the form of meat and other products from animals, many of which are fed genetically modified grains in place of omega-3-rich grasses and have been raised on antibiotics. By upping your plant protein and decreasing your animal protein, you'll drastically cut back on both of these unwelcome additions to the diet (as well as the growth-hormone residue found in the meat of many commercially raised animals, which some research suggests may be harmful).

Plant-based protein can also provide you with unique compounds shown to enrich your health—isoflavones in soy foods such as edamame, miso, and tempeh, for instance, appear to lower cholesterol, strengthen bones, and offer some protection against breast and prostate cancer.

Plant Protein Power

Below are plant foods that provide substantial protein.

- Beans (black, cannellini, kidney, pinto, chickpeas)
- Lentils (red, green, brown)
- Soy (edamame, tempeh, miso)
- Peanuts
- Nuts (almonds, walnuts, pecans, cashews, pistachios)
- Seeds (pumpkin, sunflower, sesame, chia, hemp, flax)

Protect Your Body from Oxidative Stress

A plant-based diet is also a terrific way to fortify your body with anti-oxidants, your best defense against **oxidative damage. Free radicals** are damaged, unstable molecules that are formed in manageable amounts as a natural byproduct of our metabolism—and in greater amounts when you're exposed to environmental toxins or the sun's ultraviolet rays. Free radicals hunt down other molecules to steal electrons from their cell membranes in an attempt to gain stability; this process is referred to as oxidative damage. The cell membrane, which controls what gets inside our cells and what remains outside, helps to protect our DNA—the genes that control all cell functions. When a cell is bombarded by free radicals beyond that which the body is able to handle, the cell membrane is weakened, resulting in DNA damage that changes the cell's functioning and structure. While our bodies naturally generate compounds that counteract free radicals—built-in antioxidants such as glutathione, catalase, and superoxide dismutase, for example—our systems can get overwhelmed when assaulted by too many rogue molecules. Too much oxidative damage over time exceeds the body's ability to cope and is termed **oxidative stress,** which ravages our health.

Imagine the oxidative damage that is visible on the surface of a banana or apple when exposed to the air. This is similar to the oxidative damage our cells are exposed to, which results in free radical production. And just as we can prevent the fruit from browning with the addition of lemon juice (an *anti*oxidant), so too can we prevent or lessen the damage done to our cells by choosing foods that are less inflammatory and high in antioxidants. Ideally, as free radicals bombard our cells, a plethora of phytochemicals comes to the rescue. Scores of essential nutrients found in plants offer antioxidant effects—including vitamin C (a water-soluble antioxidant that protects the watery interior of our cells), vitamin E (a fat-soluble antioxidant that protects our cell membranes, which are composed of fatty acids), selenium, and sulfur. Scientists have identified thousands of these compounds and continue to identify more, with benefits ranging from improved cardiovascular function to protection against cancer (see "Plant Power," page 233).

Increasingly linked to chronic disease, oxidative stress also speeds up aging itself on a cellular level. Research shows that oxidative stress can lead to shortening of the telomeres, structures at the end of DNA strands that safeguard our genetic material. As telomeres get shorter and shorter, cells lose their ability to divide, eventually dying off and advancing the aging process. But by keeping your body flush with anti-oxidants, you can help short-circuit oxidative stress: these selfless molecules donate electrons to free radicals (thus preventing them from going after more of your cells) and also help mend existing oxidative damage to your DNA.

Build Your Plant Base

If you're eating the SAD, shifting to a plant-based diet takes intention and commitment. While the USDA food pyramid used to recommend five to nine servings of vegetables and fruit, we advise people to be more ambitious than that and **aim for nine to eleven servings**—ideally, six to nine from vegetables and two to three from fruit. (See page 294 if you're unsure what constitutes a serving.) The best way to achieve that is to use every meal and snack as an opportunity to get a couple of servings of vegetables and fruit. Think of it as building a solid, protective foundation—your body's **plant base.** Challenge yourself: how many veggies can you eat before 4 P.M.? Hints: Chop up spinach and tomatoes and add them to scrambled eggs; eat a bed of leafy greens and curried lentils for lunch.

You can also retrofit some of your favorite dishes with some simple additions that up your dose of vegetables, fruit, and plant-based protein:

- Shred veggies—such as zucchini, carrots, or broccoli—and add them to sauces, casseroles, salads, and sandwiches.
- Substitute mashed black beans for some or all of the meat in meat loaf, meatballs, or burgers.
- Add baby spinach or other greens, such as kale, to fruit-based smoothies.

- Thicken creamy sauces and soup with silken tofu or amaranth and millet.
- Add chopped nuts to salads, oatmeal, yogurt, cookies, and casseroles, or substitute nut flours for some or all of the wheat flour in recipes.
- Put avocado slices on sandwiches and in salads, or use as a spread in lieu of mayonnaise on sandwiches; mix with eggs for a twist on egg salad.
- Add ground flaxseed (sold pre-ground as flax meal) to smoothies, yogurt, and oatmeal for a healthy dose of plant omega-3s and mixed fibers.

The more you increase your plant base, the less room there is for refined and processed foods. We talk to clients about **crowding out:** you're so busy eating the good stuff—vegetables and fruit, whole grains, and legumes—that you'll crowd out (maybe even forget about) the bad stuff.

Plant Power

Here are six key phytochemicals found to boost health and support a healthy weight:

Phytochemical: anthocyanins
How it heals: Shown to slow oxidative stress and improve blood-sugar metabolism, anthocyanins may help lower blood pressure and cholesterol. Animal research also demonstrates that they may help prevent obesity.
Where to get it: berries, pomegranates, red grapes, kidney beans

Phytochemical: indole-3-carbinol
How it heals: Preliminary research suggests that indole-3-carbinol can bring about beneficial changes in the way your body breaks down estrogen and, in turn, boost your defense against the devel-

opment of certain estrogen-sensitive cancers (such as breast cancer and cervical cancer). It is also an important source of sulfur compounds essential to support the detoxifying role of the liver.

Where to get it: cruciferous vegetables (including dark leafy greens, broccoli, cabbage, turnips, and Brussels sprouts)

Phytochemical: lignans

How it heals: A type of phytoestrogen (a class of phyto-chemicals with estrogen-like effects), lignans may help preserve bone health, reduce choles-terol, and curb the risk of breast and ovarian cancer.

Where to get it: flaxseed, pumpkin seeds, oats, beans, and berries

Phytochemical: quercetin

How it heals: In addition to dampening inflammation, quercetin appears to act as a natural anti-histamine and helps alleviate allergy symptoms. There's also evidence that quercetin can stimu-late the immune system to fend off the common cold.

Where to get it: red onions, apples, black tea, buckwheat

Phytochemical: lycopene

How it heals: Lycopene shows promise in the prevention of prostate cancer and lung cancer. Also found to fight oxidative stress, it may help lessen the risk of cardiovascular disease.

Where to get it: tomatoes, watermelon, pink grapefruit, papaya

Phytochemical: curcumin

How it heals: A powerful anti-cancer and anti-inflammatory compound, curcumin—the active ingredient in the spice turmeric—has been shown to have immense healing potential. Research suggests that it may help prevent intestinal, skin, and liver cancers and potentially stop certain cancers from progressing by triggering tumor cell death (apoptosis). It also may inhibit the buildup of amyloid beta, a substance that forms the brain plaques associated with Alzheimer's disease. Animal research suggests that, in addition, curcumin may help discourage weight gain by stalling the spread of fat tissue.

Where to get it: Turmeric is available in powdered form (and sometimes fresh) in grocery stores. It's commonly used as an ingredient in curry and can be added to soups and stir-fries.

Taking Stock

The questionnaire below, created by the Institute for Functional Medicine, can help to give you a ballpark sense of how well you're eating. As you're making changes in how you nourish your body, come back to this questionnaire to see how your score changes. (Note that some of the serving sizes differ slightly from the ones we base our recommendations on, found on page 294.)

How Healthy Is Your Diet?

Circle your answers after careful thought, then add up your points (numbers in parentheses).

1. How many fruits do you *normally* eat each day (½ cup fresh or ¼ cup dried fruit, 1 medium piece, 1 cup *unsweetened* juice)?

    A. 0 (–2)
    B. 1 (0)
    C. 2 to 3 (+2)
    D. 4 or more (+3)

    (score)_____

2. How many vegetable servings do you *normally* eat each day (1 cup leafy greens, ½ cup any other veggie, raw or cooked)?

    A. 0 (–4)
    B. 1 (0)
    C. 2 (+1)
    D. 3 (+2)
    E. 4 or more (+3)

    (score)_____

3. How many different varieties of vegetables do you eat in a normal month?

    A. 2 or less (–4)
    B. 3 to 4 (0)
    C. 5 to 6 (+1)
    D. 7 to 8 (+3)
    E. 9 or more (+4)

    (score)_____

4. How many times do you eat dried beans or peas (legumes, lentils, chickpeas, kidney beans, green peas, etc.) in a normal week?

    A. 0 (–2)
    B. 1 to 2 (0)
    C. 3 to 4 (+1)
    D. 5 to 6 (+2)
    E. 7 or more (+3)

    (score)_____

5. How many times do you eat red meat in a normal week?

    A. 6 or more (–4)

    B. 4 to 5 (–3)

    C. 1 to 3 (–1)

    D. Less than once a week (+2)

    E. 0 (+3)

                                            (score)_____

6. How many times do you eat in a fast-food restaurant in a normal week?

    A. 6 or more (–5)

    B. 4 to 5 (–4)

    C. 1 to 3 (–3)

    D. Less than once a week (–2)

    E. 0 (0)

                                            (score)_____

7. In a typical day, what do you drink *most* often?

    A. Soda (regular or diet) (–4)

    B. Caffeinated coffee or tea (–1)

    C. Decaffeinated coffee or tea (0)

    D. Milk or fruit juice (0)

    E. Herbal tea or water (+3)

                                            (score)_____

8. How many 12-ounce cans of soda do you drink in a normal day?

    A. 6 or more (–5)

    B. 4 to 5 (–4)

    C. 2 to 3 (–3)

    D. 1 (–2)

    E. Less than 1 (–1)

    F. 0 (0)

                                            (score)_____

9. How often do you eat fish in a typical week?

   A. Never (–2)
   B. Once (+1)
   C. Twice (+2)
   D. 3 to 5 times (+3)

   (score)_____

10. In a typical week, how often do you eat whole grains (100% whole-grain bread, whole oats, brown rice, quinoa, whole rye crackers)?

    A. Never (–3)
    B. 1 to 2 times a week (–1)
    C. 3 to 4 times a week (0)
    D. 5 to 6 times a week (+1)
    E. 1 or more times a day (+3)

    (score)_____

11. How often do you eat sweets such as cookies, cake, or ice cream?

    A. 1 or more times a day (–3)
    B. Every other day (–2)
    C. Twice a week (–1)
    D. Once a week (0)
    E. 2 to 3 times a month (+1)
    F. Rarely (+3)

    (score)_____

Your total score _____

Scoring:

22–28: Great eating habits

17–21: Pretty good eating habits

10–16: Needs some improvement

9 or less: Needs much improvement; try to change one habit at a time

Setting Your Intention

Understanding the powerful ways that food affects your health is one thing; putting that knowledge into practice is another. Along with practicing your mindfulness skills and creating sustainable goals, setting an intention is a powerful tool for change. You already practiced setting intention when you visualized your "best self" in chapter 1. Now you'll focus your intention on your relationship with food, so that ultimately, the majority of your choices are worthy of your best self.

We've found that how we eat is informed by what we expect from our food. For some people, food is simply "fuel" to get through the day. For others, eating is primarily about entertainment. Without judgment, give some thought to what you currently expect from food—or, stated another way, how you use food. For example:

- To celebrate
- To comfort or to be comforted
- To distract myself from other problems
- To honor my culture and traditions
- Out of necessity
- To avoid illness
- To heal
- To entertain myself when bored
- To socialize
- To get energy for day-to-day activities
- To age in the healthiest way possible
- To help protect against chronic illness

Some of our underlying expectations about food are realistic; food is a great source of energy and can help us prevent illness, for instance. Other expectations can get us into trouble. While everyone engages in comfort eating sometimes, we tend to make unhealthy choices when comfort is our *primary* expectation of food.

By setting our intention on eating in order to provide our bodies with a nourishing foundation for good health, we can begin to shift our underlying expectations of food. When this happens—when we *expect* food to support our health—choosing nourishing foods over harmful foods becomes clearer and easier.

Knowing what you now know, are you ready to set your intention on eating in a way that deeply supports your health and is worthy of your best self?

Genetics Is Not Destiny

We see a lot of patients with weight-related chronic illnesses like diabetes and heart disease, and many attribute their conditions to "bad genes." Each of us inherits thousands of genetic sequences from our parents and grandparents, some of which predispose us to certain conditions and diseases (given certain conditions or environments). However, new research shows that most of us are in no way destined to follow our parents' and grandparents' history of illness.

Overwhelming evidence in the emerging field of epigenetics demonstrates that while we all inherit genetic proclivities toward certain conditions and illnesses, how we live—including the air we breathe, the water we drink, how much we move our bodies, and what and how much we eat—affects whether those genes get expressed or not. Nutritional genomics is a specialty within epigenetics that focuses on how the foods we eat inform and instruct our DNA. Over time, these instructions have the power to keep the genes for many chronic diseases switched in the "off" position, effectively silencing them. And guess what? The wide variety of healthy, whole foods we've recommended—plant foods in particular—work to do just that. Even with a strong family history, when we optimize our biochemistry through a plant-based, whole-foods, anti-inflammatory diet, we can begin to change our destiny.

CHAPTER 11

How Much Food Do You Really Need?

"My doctor told me to stop having intimate dinners
for four. Unless there are three other people."

—Orson Welles

Just as we get conditioned to the quality of food we eat, we get used to the quantity, be it just enough or far too much. And *far too much* has become the order of the day. In restaurants and at home, portions have ballooned in the last fifty years, taking our waistlines along with them. In addition to eating supersized portions, our between-meal eating and sweetened-beverage consumption have skyrocketed. And it doesn't take much to pack on the pounds: consider that even an extra three bites per day of food may add up to 100 extra calories per day. With 365 days in a year, that is an estimated extra 10 pounds per year gained—from *three extra bites a day*. Even half of that can easily explain the weight "creep" that so many of our clients report. You may not notice an extra 5 pounds over the course of a year, but as the years and decades pass, it becomes significant. Besides having a direct, damaging effect on millions of Americans' weight and overall health, the portion explosion has distorted our perception of what is normal, leaving many people—perhaps *most* people—with no concept of what constitutes a meal's (or a day's) worth of food.

To counteract habitual overeating, we need, first and foremost, a reality check—and then a realistic plan for cutting back. In this chapter we'll focus on how to adjust your intake mindfully.

Reality Check

Eating in a way that prioritizes your health goals and cultivating in-the-moment awareness is the healthiest, most effective way to curb overeating and manage your weight for the long haul. That in-the-moment awareness reminds you to check in—*Am I hungry? Why am I eating this? How will I decide when to stop eating? Will a couple of bites of this suffice? Is this food supporting my health?*

Understanding your own body's energy needs—and how much food you take in versus how much your body uses—is one important piece of the weight management puzzle. While keeping in mind that food functions differently in each of us and provides instruction to our cells, let's consider the role of food as fuel for the body. You might remember from high-school chemistry that a calorie is the amount of energy it takes to raise a gram of water by one degree Celsius. How many calories you need depends in large part on your level of activity and your basal metabolic rate—the number of calories your particular body would require to perform the basic bodily functions if it were planted on a couch all day (just breathing, metabolizing, etc.). If you're curious, you can get a rough estimate of your rate—along with how many calories you need to maintain your current weight or lose weight—at webmd.com/diet/healthtool-metabolism-calculator. Keep in mind, though, that the formulas currently used to calculate these estimates are based on averages from huge numbers of people, and recent data show these estimates are highly inaccurate for some individuals, particularly people over forty.

While there's a lot more to weight management than a simple "calories in minus calories out" equation, in general, if you're regularly taking in more food than your body is using, you'll see your weight start to creep up, and if you regularly take in significantly less, you'll lose weight. Given that most Americans are consuming vastly more than their bodies need, and that dieting doesn't work in the long term, we need to figure out how to shift our intake in ways that are sustainable and nourishing. That starts by looking at exactly where our extra calories come from.

Culprit 1: Calorie Bombs

Shelley, age 42, came to us with a common weight-gain story. She had gained about 30 pounds since graduating from college, but had no idea how it happened. "I didn't gain it all at once," said Shelley. "It came on really slowly, so slowly I didn't even notice." Unlike many clients, she did not have a history of yo-yo dieting, and she didn't eat dessert often. But when Shelley began really tracking her diet, she realized that she fell prey to the biggest overeating culprit: calorie bombs.

Calorie bombs are another name for the gigantic portions that are far too easy to swallow: a 2,000-calorie plateful of fettuccine Alfredo from the all-you-can-eat buffet, a 350-calorie deli bagel (and that's without the cream cheese), or a 750-calorie Cobb salad. Food companies and restaurants have tapped into the American love affair with abundance and "getting a good deal." They have found creative ways to offer excessive portions of low-cost food to feed our eager palates. Pasta, bread, cheap oils, and sugar—ingredients that pack on pounds, increase inflammation, and wreak havoc on blood sugar—cost restaurants very little and keep customers coming back for more "abundance." The all-you-can-eat buffet is one giant calorie bomb. Other calorie bombs are value meals and combos, in which cheap, high-calorie drinks and fries are added to a meal for next-to-nothing cost-wise. A supersized soft drink, topping out at over 50 ounces and 600 calories, is a calorie bomb in and of itself.

But the damage isn't confined to restaurants. People quickly got used to out-to-eat portions and started filling up their plates at home with mountains of food, whether eating a vegetable stir-fry, lasagna, or a simple bowl of cereal, which was the case with Shelley, the client who had unconsciously gained 30 pounds since college. "It was granola—healthy stuff—with nuts and oats, and I always added a lot of fruit and yogurt. Then I measured it one day. Eight hundred calories! That's more than half of what my body needs for the *whole day*."

We also started adding all the restaurant extras—a nice loaf of crusty bread and extra-virgin olive oil on lasagna night, chips and salsa alongside our burritos, and, of course, dessert after every meal. Slowly but surely, supersized meals became the new normal.

Size Matters

Consider how portion sizes have grown for a few standard American diet staples. None of these foods were ever healthy, but their expanded sizes mean that they now inflict even more damage than before.

Food	1950s	Today
Hamburger	3.9 oz.	up to 12 oz.
French fries	2.4 oz.	6.7 oz.
Pasta	1.5 cups	3 cups
Bakery muffin	3 oz.	6.5 oz.
Soda	7 oz.	12 to 50 oz.

Supersized meals tend to be made up of refined foods that, consumed regularly over time, can cause inflammation. The larger the portion, the more damage that's caused. The exercise below will give you a sense of how your normal portions compare with what your body needs to maintain (or lose) weight, and how many calories you consume on an average day and in an average week. It may feel tedious, but stick with it, because the knowledge you gain is invaluable when combined with mindful eating skills and healthy-eating principles. You may never look at a bagel the same way again.

Exercise: Track Your Portions

There's only one way to know for sure how much you're eating, and that's to track your portions for a week (or longer if needed). Ideally, measure your food *after* you've plated it but *before* you eat. It's natural to eat less when you're paying attention, but remember that you're just gathering information. Try to measure what you would normally eat. Later, you'll find out how your portions compare with healthy portions. As always, cultivate kindness toward yourself. If you find yourself thinking self-critical thoughts, replace them with a neutral thought such as, "I'm just learning; now I know." You have to start somewhere. Eventually you will be able to eyeball your portions.

- *Pasta, grains, cereal, and beans/legumes.* Suppose you eat dry cereal or oatmeal in the morning, or pasta for dinner. Serve up your normal portion, and then pour it into a measuring cup.

- *Vegetables and fruit.* When possible, measure the exact quantity. But it's also fine to note "1 small banana," "1 large carrot," or "half a large apple."

- *Liquids.* For caloric beverages (anything other than water and plain tea or coffee), pour what you'd normally pour and then measure it. For milk in cereal, start by pouring 8 ounces of milk in a little pitcher and adding it to the cereal from the measuring pitcher. Keep adding measured amounts until you get to your normal portion.

- *Oils and sauces.* It's important to include often overlooked ingredients in your tracking, such as cooking oils and sauces. If you're able to pour back and measure, do so; otherwise use the technique described for milk in cereal as you're adding it to your food.

At the end of the day, calculate your total calories; online sources such as myfitnesspal.com, sparkpeople.com, or WebMD.com's "Food-o-Meter" make it easy, as packaged foods and calorie and serving amounts are listed. Be as precise as you can; don't forget that pat of butter you added to your sweet potato. What you're aiming for is a solid ballpark figure.

Be Vigilant

A lot of our clients express dismay that eating enormous portions is so easy. "Shouldn't there be some sort of stop mechanism in our bodies?" asked Kerrie, 50, one day. We actually have several stop mechanisms (see chapter 5), but in our busy, loud world, we usually override them. If our mind is off busying itself with something other than the meal we are eating (TV, computer, driving, movie, talking, etc.), we are dissociated from the act of mindful eating and likely to miss the subtle cues that suggest we stop.

Portion Plates

One strategy that makes ongoing portion tracking much easier is to make your own "portion plates" using bowls, glasses, and other serving pieces that you have in your home. Measure out typical portion sizes you are aiming for and see what dishes best fit. For example, choose a particular bowl that holds only 1 cup of cereal, a glass that holds 8 ounces of a beverage, or a bowl that holds ⅓ cup of grains.

As we discussed in chapter 5, we tend to eat nearly all the food on our plate (92 percent), regardless of the size of the plate. And afterward, we're often not aware of whether we've eaten a little or a lot. In studies, researchers offer a certain amount of a particular dish—a cup and a half of macaroni and cheese, say—and then a much larger portion of the same food on a separate occasion. Across the board, people eat significantly more when given a larger portion, up to one-third more calories. But here's the really remarkable thing: people report similar feelings of fullness despite the calorie differences—and the majority report *not noticing any difference in portion size.* In one study, for example, subjects who were served an eight-, ten-, or twelve-inch sandwich reported nearly identical ratings of fullness. The take-home message? **Cultivating your**

ability to notice subtle cues for fullness will help you feel satisfied, even with significantly smaller portions.

This phenomenon might seem like a design flaw, but it makes sense when you remember that the human body and brain have evolved for survival—which historically has meant famine rather than feast. In other words, we're better at noticing we're hungry than we are at noticing we're full. It's a little like our stress response, which turns *on* much more easily than it turns *off* in our busy twenty-first-century world. Our bodies and brains are built to respond to the occasional saber-toothed tiger and to a scarcity of food—not to unrelenting stress and unlimited access to refined carbohydrates and fats. Our biology is not a great match for the modern world, a fact that makes it all the more critical to incorporate the mindfulness skills and tools into your daily life.

Insights and Inspirations: Kris, age 39

I stopped using our regular pasta bowls—the big, wide kind—when I measured and realized they could hold more than 5 servings of pasta. I went out and bought a pretty cobalt-blue bowl about the size of my hands cupped together. I eat a lot less, just having made that simple switch.

In another 100 million years, maybe our biology will adapt. But there are ways to counteract calorie bombs in the meantime. Check out the chart on the next page to get a sense of how to eyeball healthy portions (see page 216 for our recommendations on healthy cooking methods for meat). Note that portions are not the same as serving sizes. A **serving size** is a standard amount of a type of food that is used in recommendations by consumer-health organizations and can vary depending on the source. A **portion** is the amount of food that you choose to eat at any time, which may be more or less than a serving.

Healthy Portions Cheat Sheet

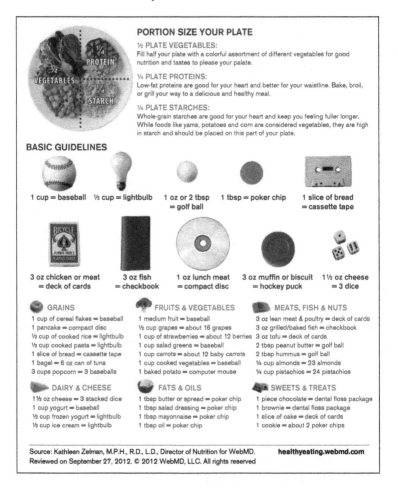

PORTION SIZE YOUR PLATE

½ PLATE VEGETABLES:
Fill half your plate with a colorful assortment of different vegetables for good nutrition and tastes to please your palate.

¼ PLATE PROTEINS:
Low-fat proteins are good for your heart and better for your waistline. Bake, broil, or grill your way to a delicious and healthy meal.

¼ PLATE STARCHES:
Whole-grain starches are good for your heart and keep you feeling fuller longer. While foods like yams, potatoes and corn are considered vegetables, they are high in starch and should be placed on this part of your plate.

BASIC GUIDELINES

- 1 cup = baseball
- ½ cup = lightbulb
- 1 oz or 2 tbsp = golf ball
- 1 tbsp = poker chip
- 1 slice of bread = cassette tape

- 3 oz chicken or meat = deck of cards
- 3 oz fish = checkbook
- 1 oz lunch meat = compact disc
- 3 oz muffin or biscuit = hockey puck
- 1½ oz cheese = 3 dice

GRAINS
- 1 cup of cereal flakes = baseball
- 1 pancake = compact disc
- ½ cup of cooked rice = lightbulb
- ½ cup cooked pasta = lightbulb
- 1 slice of bread = cassette tape
- 1 bagel = 6 oz can of tuna
- 3 cups popcorn = 3 baseballs

DAIRY & CHEESE
- 1½ oz cheese = 3 stacked dice
- 1 cup yogurt = baseball
- ½ cup frozen yogurt = lightbulb
- ½ cup ice cream = lightbulb

FRUITS & VEGETABLES
- 1 medium fruit = baseball
- ½ cup grapes = about 16 grapes
- 1 cup of strawberries = about 12 berries
- 1 cup salad greens = baseball
- 1 cup carrots = about 12 baby carrots
- 1 cup cooked vegetables = baseball
- 1 baked potato = computer mouse

FATS & OILS
- 1 tbsp butter or spread = poker chip
- 1 tbsp salad dressing = poker chip
- 1 tbsp mayonnaise = poker chip
- 1 tbsp oil = poker chip

MEATS, FISH & NUTS
- 3 oz lean meat & poultry = deck of cards
- 3 oz grilled/baked fish = checkbook
- 3 oz tofu = deck of cards
- 2 tbsp peanut butter = golf ball
- 2 tbsp hummus = golf ball
- ¼ cup almonds = 23 almonds
- ¼ cup pistachios = 24 pistachios

SWEETS & TREATS
- 1 piece chocolate = dental floss package
- 1 brownie = dental floss package
- 1 slice of cake = deck of cards
- 1 cookie = about 2 poker chips

Source: Kathleen Zelman, M.P.H., R.D., L.D., Director of Nutrition for WebMD. **healthyeating.webmd.com**
Reviewed on September 27, 2012. © 2012 WebMD, LLC. All rights reserved

A Day's Worth of Food

After scaling back her portions, one client's typical daily menu looked like this.

BREAKFAST

- 1 poached egg with 1 cup wilted spinach leaves and ½ cup asparagus
- 2 cranberry cornmeal pancakes
- 2 tsp. almond butter
- 2 tsp. maple syrup

LUNCH

- ½ cup hummus
- 1 cup mixed sliced vegetables (red pepper, carrots, celery, sugar snap peas)
- ¼ cup avocado
- 1 oz. or about 10 brown rice crackers
- 16 oz. green tea (iced)

SNACK

- 1 oz. cashews
- ½ banana

DINNER

- 4 oz. broiled salmon
- ⅓ cup quinoa
- ½ cup broccoli
- ½ cup carrots
- ¾ cup cucumber salad
- 1 tsp. olive oil
- 1 tbsp. vinegar

SNACK

- 1 cup coffee Greek yogurt with ½ cup blackberries

Calorie-Bomb Solutions

Mindful awareness. The skills you've been honing—specifically, slowing down and tuning in to your body's signals—can help you cut down on portion sizes. And simply knowing that you're likely to eat whatever portion is on your plate can prompt you to take a smaller amount in the first place.

Choose a smaller dish. The food industry uses every trick in the book to get you to eat *more,* so here are some simple "tricks" to help you eat *less.* The science is very clear on the direct relationship between the size of your plate and how much you eat. So whether you're home or at work, *use a smaller bowl or plate*! Your salad or side-dish plates can become your new dinner plates. Or dig out your grandmother's dishes—older dinnerware was much smaller. Or invest in a special bowl or plate for yourself and stick with it. If this seems too simple to work, try it for a week and see what happens.

Take it slowly. Commit to the process of slowing down your eating—no matter what it takes. Studies show that appetite-regulation hormones shift in our favor just by elongating the time spent eating a given meal. Start your meal with a meditation. Stop your meal after ten bites and check your hunger and fullness signals. Take a ten-minute break halfway through your meal before deciding if you should eat more. Consider eating with your nondominant hand, using chopsticks, or even using chopsticks with your nondominant hand! Use whatever creative ideas you have to s l o w . . . t h i n g s . . . d o w n . . .

Does your plate match your plan? Calorie bombs don't come in the form of broccoli, spinach, carrots, or lentils. It's shockingly easy to consume extra calories when you're hewing to the standard American diet. And while it is possible to eat oversized portions of healthy foods, the more you follow the principles outlined in chapter 10—in particular, choosing whole foods and combining protein, healthy fats, and slow-burning carbs (including an abundance of vegetables and fruits)—the less likely you are to overeat. Whether you're at home or eating out, ask yourself questions such as the following *at every meal:*

- What whole grains can I choose instead of more processed varieties? (Choose bulgur, quinoa, teff, or barley over white rice.)
- What extra vegetables can I add alongside my mixed greens salad?
- Where's my protein? (Think fish, lentils, nuts, cottage cheese, eggs, grass-fed beef, or free-range poultry.)
- How many servings of vegetables and whole fruit am I getting? Have I hit my nine to eleven servings? (Remember the crowding-out principle and the goal of increasing your plant base.)
- How colorful is my plate? Can I add some greens? Some blues? Some red, orange, or yellow?
- Is there some healthy fat (olive oil, avocado, nuts, seeds) on this plate?

Restaurant realities. Managing portions when eating out can be challenging, but keep the strategies above in mind, and if you eat out a lot, aim to make it work *toward* your health goals instead of against them whenever possible. Remember too that historically, eating out was a once-in-a-blue-moon event—and now many of us eat out more often than not. Knowing that there will be another restaurant adventure in your near future can help with self-restraint. You'll find additional dining-out strategies in chapter 12.

"Amorphous Foods" and Judging Portions

We have a harder time judging portions when eating foods that do not have a distinct shape, such as macaroni and cheese or mashed potatoes, and this often leads us to overeat. In general, whole foods *do* have a distinct shape and amounts are therefore easier to gauge, while also containing more fiber and bulk to fill us up. So instead of macaroni and cheese, eat brown rice with beans and vegetables. And instead of mashed potatoes, eat a small baked potato with the skin, plus some fish and greens. When you do eat "amorphous" foods, keep in mind that your perception may be skewed, and try eating half of what's on your plate. Be open to when a taste of something may be enough.

The "just a taste" strategy can also be helpful for pasta. Because pasta is inexpensive, cooks up quickly at the end of a long day, and we all love it, it has become a staple for many people. But that means dinner, too often, is white flour on a plate. Pasta is better served up as an accent—primavera-style with a gorgeous grouping of vegetables or black beans, with lots of garlic and seasonings.

Culprit 2: Snacking and Grazing

Eating and drinking between meals now accounts for an average of 25 percent of daily calories, according to surveys. In fact, some studies suggest that our collective excess calories—and excess weight—now come more from snacking than from oversized portions.

This makes a lot of sense, given the trends in our culture. Processed snack foods—and images of these foods through advertising—have vastly increased. Given our brain's default—to eat the food we see, if it's enticing—it's not surprising that our between-meal nibbling has increased as well.

Don't get us wrong: food eaten between meals *can* be a nutritious part of a healthy diet, and research shows that eating five or six "mini-meals" can be an effective approach to weight management by boosting metabolism and stabilizing blood sugar. People get into trouble, though, when they add healthy snacks but don't adjust the size of their main meals. And there's nothing healthy about snacking on chips and other processed foods. By and large, these foods add calories, unhealthy carbohydrates and fats, and chemical additives—but very little in the way of nutrients or fiber. Remember your *intention*; unhealthy snacks represent a missed opportunity to give your body something that it does need.

A subset of snacking, **grazing,** is just what it sounds like: the chips you munch on while finishing a report at work, the nibbling you do while preparing dinner, the Jordan almonds you grab from a colleague's candy bowl, the last few bites of your son's peanut-butter sandwich that you scarf down not because you're hungry, but because you hate throwing food away. Grazing is the epitome of mindless eating, because we hardly realize we're doing it. It's easy to take in a shocking number of calories from continuous munching and to hardly notice you're doing so.

"Between pre-dinner nibbling and the ubiquitous chips and cookies at the office, I was eating about a thousand calories from snacking. A thousand!" said Shelley, after spending a week tracking her calories. "And then three big meals on top of that." That's not unusual. We are bad at gauging the amount of food we've eaten, especially when we're not paying attention. Mindfulness helps.

Exercise: Track Your Snacks

Spend a week noting all your between-meal eating. Don't worry about calorie counts; just write down what you eat, how much, and when. (Examples: Handful of potato chips while standing at a coworker's desk before lunch, jelly beans left over from kids' Easter basket while making dinner.) At the end of the week, tally your between-meal snacks, including calories if you wish. Did the amount surprise you? What situations or environments were triggers for between-meal eating? And what do you think you really needed at each of those times? Were you bored, tired, or truly hungry? Make notes and observe where there is opportunity to change your behavior.

Snacking and Grazing Solutions

Make snacking count. The most important thing to remember is that snacks *matter*, in terms of calories and nutrition, just as much as meals do. If you find that you need to eat more frequently than three meals per day, change your mind-set. Instead of thinking of your daily eating plan as three meals and a snack or two, intentionally adjust your portions so that you eat five or six mini-meals, each with a balance of lean protein, slow-burning carbohydrates, and healthy fat. Further, consider each mini-meal as an opportunity to get a few servings of veggies or fruit.

Graze like a cow—on plants. If you get the munchies while making dinner or working on a deadline, remember that you have a choice about what to munch on. Take your cue from nature's true grazers, cows, and graze on plants. Be sure to set up your environment in a way that supports this intention: keep cut-up celery, carrots, sugar snap peas, and other vegetables in the fridge (and at work if possible) for the express purpose of grazing.

Mindful awareness. Snacking and grazing are especially prone to mindlessness. We are creatures of habit, living in a culture in which food is everywhere. Bring your awareness to your body sensations, thoughts, and emotions—and to your environment—with simple but powerful questions: *Why am I eating this food? Because it's there? Am I bored? Am I actually hungry? If so, what's a healthy choice? What's going to make my body feel good?* In the chain analysis process you practiced in chapter 9, you learned that you have the power to make choices before an eating episode spirals out of control. If you do decide to eat a snack food like chips or cookies, for instance, you now know that you *can* eat just a few bites. Remember that small amounts of these foods are just as satisfying as large ones. Be mindful of the "clean plate club" fallacy, especially with snack foods. There is nothing wrong with leaving behind or throwing away unhealthy food.

Culprit 3: Stealth Calories

Stealth calories come from foods and drinks that pack a surprising punch. Sweetened beverages fall into this category because it is *so very easy* to slurp them down quickly, and Americans have been doing so more and more over the last twenty years.

Like other fast-burning carbs, sugary drinks send our blood sugar on a wild ride, and as we've discussed, beverages are especially insidious because our bodies do not seem to register "liquid calories" in the same way they do calories from food. While we have a tendency to compensate for overeating solid foods by eating less food later, this is not the case for sweetened beverages. This may be because drinks don't trigger feelings of fullness or satisfaction in the way that solid food does. Sweetened drinks are the epitome of extra, empty calories.

Artificially sweetened soft drinks are equally problematic, and potentially more so, for reasons scientists are just beginning to understand. They don't contain calories but are still linked to overeating and weight gain. Alcoholic drinks, too, can be a double whammy in terms of calorie intake; they contain significant calories themselves and also increase overeating, in part by compromising our discernment and lowering our inhibitions.

Foods made up of refined, processed carbohydrates are another form of stealth calories. Pasta, bagels, chips, baked goods, and packaged snacks contain more calories per square inch than the vast majority of whole foods do, with less fiber and bulk. So even if you don't eat a large portion of refined carbs, you're probably taking in more calories than you think. And foods that are calorie-packed but low in fiber and other nutrients tend to not fill you up. That's why you can eat a giant bowl of pasta or half a bag of Goldfish or potato chips and still feel hungry. Fiber, abundant in vegetables, whole grains, and fruit, is instrumental in fullness and satiety, as is protein.

Healthy fats play an important role in satisfaction and fullness, but it's important to be aware that *all* fats are rich in calories and easy to overdo. In the "healthy-but-stealthy" category: olive oil, at 120 calories a tablespoon, and nuts, at 160 calories per quarter cup. Unhealthy fats, of course, are rich in calories, too. Restaurants use copious amounts of oil and butter to make creamy, decadent sauces and other dishes, and packaged and prepared foods are often loaded with unhealthy oils and shortening. Salads, an ostensibly healthy choice, can weigh in at more than 700 calories when they're drenched in oil-laden dressings and high-fat toppings.

Stealth Calorie Solutions

Limit your liquid calories. Water should be the primary beverage you consume, with a few exceptions, such as green, black, and herbal teas and small amounts of antioxidant-rich juices such as tart cherry, pomegranate, and blueberry. If you drink sweetened or diet beverages, gradually cut back. If you don't like the taste of water, add slices of citrus or a splash of juice, preferably one of those mentioned above. If you love carbonation, try sparkling water. Be sure to give your body and taste buds time to adjust to the more interesting and less sweet taste of some of these beverages before deciding how often to have them.

Come back to your core healthy eating principles. Eat to nourish your body. Forget about the candy bar. A small portion of *whole* grains (think barley, quinoa, teff, black rice, or brown rice) with vegetables and fish, besides being good for all-around health and disease prevention, will satisfy and fill you up. It's the diet that our bodies evolved to eat that is most healthy and sustainable.

Be conscious of fats. If you tend to put butter on everything, see what it's like to use half the usual amount, and then after a week or so, half of that. Even better, try using a small amount of extra-virgin olive oil, coconut oil, or other healthy fat. If you use fat to add flavor, experiment with fresh herbs and spices and aromatic vegetables such as garlic, spring onions, or roasted peppers. Instead of drenching your salad in creamy dressing, add accompaniments like fresh berries and/or a small amount of high-flavor cheese such as goat or feta, and experiment with flavor-infused vinegar.

Prepare your own food. Restaurants specialize in stealth calories. The creamy sauces, abundant bread and butter, and enticing cocktails are all jam-packed with calories. In the next chapter, you'll learn more about how to integrate more home cooking into your routine. In the meantime, politely ask how foods are prepared, and speak up if you want sauces and dressings on the side.

Cutting Back: Slow and Steady . . . It's Not a Race

Becoming aware of how many calories you've been taking in can throw you for a loop. "I realized I was eating an average of 3,000 calories a day. On days when I had business lunches or dinners, I was easily consuming more than 4,000 calories," said Shelley. But remember that what you've gained is information, pure and simple. Now you get to decide what to do with it.

Realizing that your usual bowl of breakfast cereal is a whopping 700 calories may come as a shock, but cutting it in half may be shocking in its own right, to both your mind and your stomach. Resist the urge to slash calories suddenly and drastically, because that often backfires. **Eating too few calories a day causes metabolic changes that can make your body hold on to weight.** Slow and steady wins the race; start by revamping one meal at a time, or one particularly challenging snack.

Research shows that people who are trying to lose weight tolerate cutting out between 100 and 500 calories a day without much struggle. This may very well happen by focusing on the culprits and solutions in this chapter, and by coming back to the principles in chapter 10, in particular eating whole foods and being sure to get a balance of protein, healthy carbs, and healthy fat every time you eat. We also like to emphasize "low-hanging fruit," the stuff in your diet that's *easiest* to cut out or modify. For one client, Jeanine, who was eating about 2,200 calories a day, we looked for low-hanging fruit and found plenty. She often ordered salads for lunch but started asking for dressing on the side; she found she used only half the dressing and didn't miss the rest (saving 150 calories). When she ate sandwiches, she started using just one slice of bread—open-faced instead of traditional. She found that she enjoyed the sour taste of plain yogurt just as well as the sweetened kind, which saved her about 60 calories per serving. With simple changes like this, she cut about 300 calories from her daily diet—and didn't miss them. Consider the modifications below; then fill in your own.

Excess calories	Modification
Margarita (500 calories)	12-ounce beer (150 calories)
Two slices of bread (220 calories)	Brown rice tortilla (130 calories)
Mocha latte (330 calories)	Coffee with milk (25 calories) and a dash of cinnamon
_____	_____
_____	_____
_____	_____
_____	_____

Timing Is Everything (or at Least, It's Something)

Paying attention to *when* you eat can help you control what and how much you eat. The jury is still out on whether calories eaten at different times of day have different effects on our weight and metabolism. However, a few recent studies suggest that there may be some truth to the dieting maxim that eating at night affects metabolism differently than eating during the day and can therefore contribute to excessive insulin levels and weight gain. Setting aside the effects of particular times of day on metabolism, here's how timing can absolutely affect your food intake—quantity and quality—and consequently your weight and health.

It's common to "backload" eating, meaning that we take in most of our calories in the late afternoon and evening. Here's what happens: for any number of reasons, we eat little or no breakfast and then don't eat well during the day due to work demands and stress. By dinnertime, we're extremely hungry and relieved to be done with the day, and we might feel that we *deserve* to indulge a little. We overdo it at dinner, with calorie-laden pasta and other starches, rich food, and dessert. If we have a partner and/or children, this may be our first chance to connect with them in a relaxed manner. So what happens? We sit and eat, talk and eat, laugh and eat, and keep eating. Over time this becomes the new normal, and that glass of wine or dessert that used to be for a special occasion is now an expectation.

Insights and Inspirations: Erica, age 38

I've never been a breakfast person, and then by the time I get to work, I'm jazzed up on coffee, which kills my appetite. I grab a salad at lunch and eat it at my desk. Then I get home, and anything goes. I'm usually ravenous, so I'll eat cheese and crackers or chips and salsa when I'm cooking. Then dinner ends up being a big bowl of linguine and whatever else we're having. And dessert, that's a nightly staple. When I tracked my food intake I realized I was eating about 3,500 calories a day on weekdays and that I had nearly 75 percent of those calories from 4 P.M. to 10 P.M. This shocked me! On the weekends, when I ate more food (and healthier food) earlier in the day, I ate less overall.

If you suspect you're a "backloader," start intentionally shifting your habits so that your calories are evenly distributed throughout the day. Start with breakfast—meaning, first and foremost, *eat one* (preferably a high-protein one). This is the one instance in *The Mindful Diet* in which we'll encourage you to eat even if you're not hungry. Eventually, you'll experience a desire to eat in the morning. Research shows that people who skip breakfast are at higher risk of obesity and that eating breakfast encourages making healthier food choices throughout the day. Biochemically, this makes sense. Your morning meal is "breaking the fast." When you prolong that fast by skipping it, this increases your body's insulin response when you do eat, which in turn can increase your body's fat storage and eventually lead to weight gain. We also know that those individuals who are successful at maintaining significant weight loss report eating breakfast regularly.

Equally important is what you eat for breakfast. In our culture, breakfast is often a bowl or plateful of refined carbohydrates: cereal, toast, bagels, Danishes. That means we're starting the day with a blood-sugar rush—which, as we explained in chapter 10, begets a crash and subsequent rush, and another, and another. Try rethinking your breakfast as a meal like any other instead of a set of specialized foods. Some cultures have breakfasts that resemble lunch or dinner—and often are leftovers from the previous day's meal. In Israel, breakfast often includes chopped salad with smoked fish; in Barcelona, salmon, capers, cheeses, and meats. In Costa Rica, a dish called *gallo pinto*—rice, beans, and often eggs—is a common morning meal. So begin to ask yourself, "What else is possible?" At a minimum, combine slow-burning carbs (vegetables, fruit, or whole grains), a lean protein, and a healthy fat choice. The next chapter has mix-and-match charts to get you started.

For many people, breaking the three-meals-a-day paradigm can help as well. Eating five or six mini-meals instead can help you stabilize your blood-sugar and insulin levels and stay "ahead of the crash." But remember, this strategy works only when amounts are small.

Beyond the Numbers

The most important part of the reality check, more important than calorie numbers and portion sizes, is a reminder of the basic fact that the purpose of food is *to nourish our bodies, support our health, and give us energy*. While it is fine for food to be one source of pleasure and part of our social traditions, our culture has lost sight of its essential purpose. As you've learned, people use food for many other things—to distract, to comfort, as a constant source of pleasure or stimulation—and food companies manipulate food and use it to make money. Manufacturers have worked for many years to come up with just the right combinations of ingredients to redefine the purpose of eating. In this paradigm, food is for buying and eating: buy, open, eat, repeat.

Coming back to the true purpose of food and your intention when choosing what to eat can be very powerful. Asking yourself simple questions can help you make choices—at the grocery store, in your kitchen, at the dining room table, at restaurants—about not only what to eat, but how much: *What is this food for? What foods does my body need? How much does my body need?*

When Shelley began cutting back, she realized that her body needed a lot less food than she'd been giving it. "I was constantly 'on'—always on the computer or on the phone with clients at work, and then busy with my kids at home," she says. "It was almost like food had become another source of stimulation. I was totally disconnected from its purpose for my body." When she started reconnecting with that purpose—wanting to give her body the nutrients and calories it needed without overloading it—the effects were profound. "I had to really stop and think, 'What is this food for? Is this what my body needs? Am I going for quality here, or just quantity?'" she says. After a while, eating "just enough"—and choosing nutritious food—became second nature.

Whoopie-Pie Moments

Treats—sweet or savory—can and should be an integral part of a healthy eating plan, even when you are trying to cut back. The problem, of course, is that the whole concept of a treat has lost its meaning. Junky, sugary foods are ubiquitous; there's nothing special about them in either quality or quantity. Children, who are a pure reflection of our food culture, ask for (and often get) treats every day, and sometimes multiple times a day. Social and family-related gatherings can lead to treat overload due to excitement, anxiety, habit, or others' expectations (think well-intentioned relatives pushing cookies on everyone who enters the house). And many of us are used to reaching for treats out of habit or to fill emotional needs.

By considering our true needs and finding ways to meet them without relying on food, we can **redefine our rewards.**

Still, it's worth coming back to the concept behind the word "treat": special food for a special occasion. In our practice, we talk to clients about "whoopie-pie moments," a term inspired by Mary, a beloved babysitter Beth had as a child. As the world's best babysitter, Mary knew how to do all kinds of magical things, including making whoopie pies. When Mary died in her twenties from breast cancer, her whoopie-pie recipe became a symbol of love and "everything Mary" for Beth and her family. Whoopie-pie moments speak to the emotions that are deeply tied to certain foods we eat—and moments we share with people. They are occasional, very special, and thoroughly enjoyed indulgences. Your whoopie-pie moment might be eating a butterscotch sundae on your annual trip to see your best friend from childhood, because that's what you used to eat together as teenagers. Or it might be having a decadent meal out at a French restaurant once a month with your husband, or sharing some of your favorite dark chocolate with colleagues to celebrate finishing a project at work.

Exercise: Creating Whoopie-Pie Moments

Mindful awareness and planning can help you shift your attitude and habits away from everyday "treats" and toward whoopie-pie moments.

1. Start by thinking about your current patterns with treats. How do you treat yourself? What are your favorite indulgences? Are treats a daily occurrence? Weekly? Do they feel special or routine? How much do you enjoy your treats? Is there ever guilt or self-reproach involved? Are you sometimes meeting needs that are not food-related?

2. If you are meeting emotional needs with treats, think of some ways to redefine your rewards and meet your true needs.

3. To shift your attitude and habits, think about the food or foods that are truly special for you. It might be something from your childhood, like your aunt's amazing coconut cake, or it might be an adult discovery, like decadent French cheese or dark chocolate with sea salt.

4. Now think about the situations that are truly special and worthy of a food-related indulgence. Occasional dinner dates with your spouse? Visits with old friends? Celebrations for reaching personal goals? How often will these events occur? There's no wrong answer—it might be every few days, once a week, once a month, or a few times a year.

5. Not every whoopie-pie moment is planned, of course. Healthy eating does allow for spontaneity. Here are some questions to ask yourself in the moment when contemplating a treat:

   • What do I really need in this moment?

   • Is this food worthy of me?

   • Does eating this right now support my intention, my values?

   • How much of this do I need to be satisfied? (It might be less than you think.) What is "just enough"?

Allowing for joyful indulgences in your eating plan takes away the guilt of "cheating," as well as the attendant backlash. A reminder from chapter 3: When we impose rigid rules, we usually fail to follow them—that's human nature. Mentally punishing ourselves for "falling off the wagon" tends to make us spiral away from guidelines altogether, even healthy ones, in an attempt to avoid further punishment. There is nothing wrong with using food to show love, for someone else or for ourselves. It's what we do to nurture—and it is often an intensely personal way that we nourish ourselves and those we love. But it's important that it is just one way among many to "nourish" and that we do it consciously, making sure the food is *worthy* of the attention—and that it's part of an overall diet that supports our health and well-being.

CHAPTER 12

Reconnecting with Your Food

"No yoga exercise, no meditation in a chapel filled
with music will rid you of your blues better than
the humble task of making your own bread."

—M. F. K. Fisher

Successfully changing eating habits means reconnecting with our food—or perhaps connecting for the first time. Packaged foods allow us to spend minimal time in the kitchen. Despite the convenience of these foods—and the business models of several national weight-loss brands—healthy eating, for the most part, can't be done via frozen dinners, packaged meals, or takeout. Not only do processed and restaurant foods contain sky-high amounts of things that are not great for you—the sodium, trans fats, chemical additives and preservatives, and refined flours and sugars we discussed in chapter 10—but it's difficult to feel connected to anything that comes encased in plastic. When we lose a connection to our food, we lose an ability to appreciate it. And when we don't appreciate our food, we don't want to invest any time or money in it. The result is a downward spiral of choosing ever-more-convenient packaged foods, just so we don't have to think about cooking. Our health and well-being spiral downward along the way.

Cooking and preparing your own food is one of the most powerful things you can do to take charge of your health, change your relationship with food for good, and manage your weight. It's the only way to know and control exactly what you're putting in your body. Instead of relying on food manufacturers or diet trends to decide what to eat, imag-

Insights and Inspirations: Steve, age 64

For years, I ate anything I wanted, and as much of it as I could consume. I especially loved the fast-food breakfasts, any salty chip, and frozen stuffed-crust pizzas. Whenever I inevitably started noticing my pants not fitting, I'd pretty much stop eating, cutting back to only one meal a day. I thought I had the best of both worlds—I ate whatever until I gained a lot of weight, then I paid my penance and dropped back down. Then I started having less-than-perfect medical checkups. I was "on fire," as my doctor put it. Common markers of inflammation were elevated and a number of other labs began to shift. My doctor told me that if things didn't change, I would have to go on medication to control my blood pressure and blood sugar. I knew my family history, and I guess I figured it was my destiny, but the doctor said that if I changed my diet I could essentially change my future. I knew then that I had to make peace with what I ate. All of a sudden I couldn't grab food out of the freezer and be stuffed ten minutes later. It took a little while to figure out how to navigate my way around the produce aisles and my own kitchen. But now I've got a pretty good repertoire of dishes—turns out I love to make and eat soup. I even found a way to lighten up my favorite clam chowder! I cook up a big pot on Sunday afternoons and eat it all week. Most important, I feel as if I have found a rhythm that I have settled into with my diet—and I'm comfortable, at ease really for the first time in a long time. And the interesting part is that my weight doesn't yo-yo, and I'm off the cycle of bingeing and fasting. My doctor says she's proud of me, but that's nothing compared to how good I feel about myself.

ine gaining an intimate knowledge of what satisfies your taste buds and keeps your body feeling good and functioning well—along with the skills to implement that knowledge. We have seen patients transform their lives—and their health—simply by learning their way around a kitchen.

We can't promise that you'll relish every minute you spend chopping, washing, or sautéing, but we *can* promise you'll feel an increased sense of satisfaction when you master a few basic skills that empower you to make the majority of your own meals. If you embrace them, the tasks of planning your meals, choosing your ingredients, and cooking your food can be a rewarding, relaxing, and even joyful activity. If done with mindfulness, these habits will definitely change your life.

Don't panic—we're not saying that you can't use *any* prepared foods, ever. There are now a selection of packaged foods that are relatively healthy. But in order to truly know and appreciate what you're feeding your body, the majority of your diet should be whole foods that you prepare yourself.

Step 1: Get Your Head in the Game

The thought of cooking sparks strong feelings in a lot of people—fear and dread among them. Let's take a moment to examine some popular beliefs about preparing your own food, including:

- **Belief 1: It takes too much time.** Preparing your own food does indeed take time. Just a couple of generations ago, people spent the better part of their day preparing for the dinner meal. That's not possible for most people today. Planning your menus, shopping for ingredients, chopping, cooking, and cleaning up don't happen by magic, after all. *Your* time and *your* energy are required. But that doesn't mean *all* of your time and energy. You may be asking yourself, "How is this possible?" The time has to come from somewhere. The key is to prioritize cooking so that you spend time on it first, *before* you while away the evening watching *The Bachelorette* or your Sunday afternoon cruising the racks at T.J. Maxx. It's the same as budgeting your money—if you wait until the end of the month to put money into savings, you'll probably never have money "left over." But if you put a certain amount in savings as soon as you get paid, the nonvital spending will get crowded out naturally, and your savings will grow without you even having to think about where the money will come from. With the right resources, information, planning, and preparation, making tasty, delicious meals doesn't have to consume your whole day. It takes practice, like everything else, but you'll find that it becomes second nature. Think about the time you use to plan and prepare food as an investment in your health and well-being. What better investment is there?

- **Belief 2: It's a pain.** We need to eat multiple times a day, and it can be daunting to think of preparing all that food, day in and day out. Yet when you embrace cooking as a natural part of life, preparing your own food offers so many rewards. First, cooking is a creative act, one that involves all your senses and results in a product you can eat that in turn gives you the energy and nutrients you need to thrive. Preparing food is also an excellent opportunity to practice mindfulness. When you savor the aromas, feel the textures of the food, hear the sizzle as the garlic hits the pan, and prepare a plate that's pleasing to your eye, you are in the present moment. Cooking also connects you to the web of life. You enjoy a direct link to the farmers who grew the food, the drivers who transported it, the grocers who sold it, and the clerks who bagged it. It also gives you a tangible means of nourishing yourself and your family. In short, cooking (even short-order, no-frills cooking) makes life richer.

- **Belief 3: I can't cook!** We hear this again and again. "I'm a mess in the kitchen," people say. Or, "Cooking's not for me." Or, "I can boil water—that's about it." Feelings of ineptitude in the kitchen come from a variety of places: the recent focus on culinary skills on shows such as *Top Chef*; a lifetime of eating pre-packaged foods; the rising availability of takeout and prepared foods (even drugstores are beginning to stock premade sandwiches and salads); and time-crunched schedules. For women in particular, the subject of cooking can be loaded. Women have traditionally been responsible for preparing the family food, which for some people increases feelings of incompetence in the kitchen; better to avoid the subject altogether and serve hot dogs than tackle the huge mountain of knowledge that we imagine we need in order to cook. For others, it's a defensive move—if you can't cook, you also can't be tied to the kitchen night after night. Our response to all that? It takes only a handful of techniques to make an unlimited number of dishes. And the more comfortable you get in the kitchen, the easier it will be to expand your repertoire over time—no culinary school required.

- **Belief 4: I know how to cook, but the food I make doesn't taste good.** Perhaps you had an unfortunate experience with a soup you spent all afternoon on that wound up having no flavor, or a quinoa dish that tasted terrible, or an elaborate meal you made that the kids refused to touch. While every cook will have some misses once in a while, there are a few simple, healthy techniques that provide nearly universal good results. For instance, there is little that extra-virgin olive oil, garlic, and a splash of balsamic vinegar can't make tantalizing. And a smidge of sea salt and a squeeze of lemon added just before eating brings almost every dish to life. Below, we'll describe how to use simple cooking techniques, such as roasting, to bring out the flavor of food. If you've been eating primarily processed foods, with the artificial flavors, sodium, and chemicals designed to improve their flavor and mouthfeel, whole foods may taste a little flat at first. Using simple cooking techniques that brighten the flavor of real food will help your taste buds be excited about the switch. And your taste buds *will* change. In our experience, it usually takes two to four weeks to transition from processed food.

- **Belief 5: I'll end up wasting a lot of food.** Many of us have had the experience of buying a ton of produce at the store on impulse because we suddenly decide to eat more healthfully, only to have it morph into a science project at the bottom of the crisper drawer. Or the package of chicken breasts we bought on sale that we didn't cook before it went bad. Here's a tip to ensure that the food you buy at the store doesn't go to waste: start each meal prep by looking in the fridge and in your countertop bowl of produce to see what needs to be used soon *before* you decide what you'll make. It sounds obvious, but it makes a big difference. Similarly, try to buy only what you have a *plan* for that week.

- **Belief 6: I'll eat too much.** If you're increasing your exposure to food—washing, chopping, stirring, seasoning—won't you also munch your way through your meal prep and up your total caloric intake? Or, if you're cooking up big batches of food, won't you be tempted to overeat? Keeping your mindfulness practice going will help with this—staying aware of your body's signals to determine your level of hunger. If you find that you're genuinely hungry, eating a healthy snack before cooking is an option. In general, the nature of plant-based, whole-foods cooking will mean that if you *do* nosh while cooking, it'll be the carrots you're chopping instead of a bag of chips. And having a big pot of leftovers in the fridge also means you'll have a healthy alternative to reach for when you're famished and most likely to eat whatever's easiest. If *quantity* control is an issue, you can store meal-sized portions in the fridge or freezer.

Exercise: What Does Cooking Stir Up for You?

We've listed some common beliefs about cooking, but what ideas and feelings are you carrying around about it? This exercise will help you see the beliefs you hold that may be coloring your attitude toward cooking. Since you can't change a belief you don't know you have, putting your true thoughts down on paper so you can see them objectively can help clear any mental roadblocks you may have to feeling competent—and even inspired—in the kitchen. You'll need a quiet place, a pen and paper, and about fifteen minutes.

1. Sit, close your eyes, and take a few breaths, resting your attention on how the breath rises and falls in your body. Once you're in a quieter mental space, imagine yourself sitting down to write a grocery list. What thoughts come up when you do so? What emotions come up? Any sensations?

2. Now see yourself in the grocery store. What thoughts, emotions, or sensations arise? Write them down.

3. Next, imagine yourself in your kitchen, just before you're about to cook a meal—you're opening the fridge or the cabinets, deciding what to have. What are you experiencing as you imagine it? Write down the thoughts, feelings, and sensations you notice.

4. Now see yourself at the stove or cutting board. How are you feeling about the act of food preparation? Again, write it all down.

5. Finally, imagine yourself eating a plate of food you've prepared yourself. How does it taste? How are you feeling as you eat it?

Once you've completed the exercise, take a few minutes to read back through your answers. What do you notice? What insight do you have about your relationship to cooking? What part of the process elicits the most negative reaction? What parts do you enjoy? If you have a negative reaction to any parts, brainstorm a few ways to make them more palatable. How could you encourage yourself to experiment with the process?

Insights and Inspirations: Susan, age 65

Trust me when I say I was not a cook. I existed mostly on frozen dinners, canned soups, cereal, and lots and lots of ice cream. When I started having stomach problems after having my gallbladder removed, I worked with an integrative nutritionist to change my diet. At first I was very intimidated to learn how to cook whole grains and vegetables. But my gut just wasn't tolerating my old ways of eating anymore, so I stuck with it—now I'm even confident enough to invite my grown kids over for dinner. I know I can serve them (and my grandkids) something that's tasty and good for them, and that won't take me all day to prepare. I even look forward to my time in the kitchen. Much to my surprise, I've found that I do some of my best thinking when I'm standing at the stove.

Step 2: Set Yourself Up for Success

Nothing sets you up for healthy eating like being prepared. Remember, we eat what we see, both in the outside world and at home. Studies have consistently shown that foods placed on the middle shelves in grocery stores outsell items on the outskirts of the display area. Similar results are found at home. Researchers at Cornell University have found that we are three times more likely to eat the first thing we see when we look in the fridge or the cupboards than the fifth (or tenth) thing we see. To set yourself up for success, then, it's vital to shop with a plan, and then prep and store your groceries with intention once you get them home. Although these steps take time and forethought, once they're done, you'll have everything you need at your fingertips to eat for total health.

What to Toss

We'll start by clearing some shelf space and removing temptation by taking stock of what's currently in your kitchen and throwing out anything that doesn't pass muster. You can't cook food that's good for you with bad-for-you ingredients.

- **Anything containing high-fructose corn syrup.** As with any sugar, HFCS causes blood-sugar levels to spike and then crash, triggering a craving for more sugary foods. As you've learned, HFCS appears to play a role in accelerated weight gain—particularly in the form of belly fat, which is associated with a higher risk of chronic disease such as heart disease and diabetes. It is best to eradicate this particular form of sugar from your diet altogether. This requires vigilance, as HFCS shows up in all kinds of places.

  Common culprits:
  - Sodas
  - Fruit drinks
  - Sports drinks
  - Packaged baked goods
  - Cookies

- Crackers
- Sauces
- Dressings

- **Anything containing partially hydrogenated oil.** Also known as trans fats, hydrogenated oils have been chemically modified to remain solid at room temperature, meaning they help processed foods seem fresher longer. As you know, trans fats contribute to a host of negative side effects, increasing inflammation and raising levels of bad cholesterol and fats known as triglycerides—all of which are associated with increased risk of heart disease, clogged arteries, and diabetes. While trans fats are being phased out of the food supply, take time to carefully read all the labels on the food you have on hand—if you see the word "hydrogenated," toss it.

  Common culprits:
  - Margarine
  - Cookies
  - Crackers
  - Cakes
  - Granola bars

- **White flour, and anything containing white flour.** White flour is made from whole-wheat grains that have had their fibrous outer layer removed, leaving the starchy center to be bleached and processed. There is very little nutritional value left by the time the processing is through. With none of the outer layer, white flour hits the bloodstream quickly, causing a blood-sugar spike and subsequent crash. The result? You quickly crave more starchy, sugary foods to get blood-sugar levels back up; this makes you likely to overeat. On ingredient lists, white flour is listed as "wheat flour"; unless you see "*whole* wheat flour," it's from refined grains. Get off the roller coaster by discarding all the white flour and white-flour products in your pantry. You'll be sparing yourself a host of ills by doing away with them.

  Common culprits:
  - White bread
  - Pasta
  - Crackers

- Breakfast cereals
- Pretzels and other snacks
- Baked goods

- **Sodas and other presweetened beverages.** These drinks are typically loaded with HFCS—containing as much as 13 teaspoons of the sweetener in a single 12-ounce can. There's no room for soda in a healthy diet. Sweetened beverages such as iced tea, lemonade, and fruit juice–based drinks aren't much better. Consider these once-in-a-blue-moon items. The American Heart Association recommends that women consume not more than 6 teaspoons of sugar per day, and men not more than 9 teaspoons per day. That means 24 grams of sugar for women, and 36 for men. How many grams of sugar are you getting from one serving of these beverages? A 12-ounce can of Coke contains 39 grams. It's time for them to go.

- **"Binge foods."** We all have one: a food we just can't resist. For some it's a sweet treat, such as cookies; for others it's something crunchy and salty, such as chips. Whatever it is, once you start eating this food, it's hard to stop until it's all gone. We know you likely live with others who may or may not share your devotion to eating real food. But if there's something you buy "for the kids" that *you* end up eating most of, toss it.

  Common culprits:
  - Potato chips
  - Tortilla chips
  - Cookies
  - Pretzels
  - Salty snacks (e.g., Goldfish)

- **Unhealthy oils.** In order to ensure that you eat only healthy, anti-inflammatory fats, toss the following cooking oils so you won't be tempted to reach for them in a pinch:

  Soy, corn, and vegetable oil. Corn oil and soybean oil are both high in omega-6 fatty acids. Most generically termed vegetable oils are a random mix of oils; these oils leave too much mystery.

Vegetable shortenings. These are typically made with partially hy-drogenated oils, meaning they are chock-full of trans fats—the most pernicious form of fat there is.

Expired oils. Most oil goes rancid within a year; toss oils if you don't remember when you bought them or if they smell like linseed oil (paint thinner).

Chemically extracted oils. In addition to their other ills, many of the most commonly available oils—including soybean, corn, peanut, and vegetable—are extracted using hexane. This chemical is de-rived from petroleum and is also used as a solvent and a cleaning agent. Unless the oil says "cold-pressed" or "expeller-pressed" on the label, it's probably chemically extracted.

Insights and Inspirations: Carolyn, age 54

I always thought my husband and I ate fairly well; I attributed our weight gain to just another side effect of aging. But when I went through our pantry and freezer and looked at what we'd been eat-ing, I was shocked to find that most of our staples had hydrogenated oils or high-fructose corn syrup in them—or both! I thought because we didn't eat dessert all that often that we were doing really well by avoiding all that sugar. Boy, was I wrong.

Let go of whatever beliefs you've absorbed over the years about not wasting food, and toss whatever contains these ingredients. This is a one-time clean out and you are moving forward. If you are having trouble, remind yourself that *if it's there, you'll eat it—and if it's not, you won't.* It's really that simple.

What to Keep or Buy

We don't want you to end up like Old Mother Hubbard, with nothing in her cupboards. Here are the items you should keep in stock, or add to your future grocery store lists. With these key players on hand, you'll be able to create many healthy meals.

Whole grains and whole-grain products. In lieu of nutrient-lacking refined flour and products made from it, stock whole-grain versions. These include the intact grains themselves, such as brown rice, steel-cut oatmeal, buckwheat, teff, quinoa, and barley, as well as products made out of them, such as brown rice cakes, whole-wheat flour and other whole-grain flours, quinoa pasta, and buckwheat pancake mix. Look for the word "whole" in front of all "wheat" items on the ingredient list—merely opting for "multi-grain" is no guarantee that those grains are unrefined. See "Eat Like an Ancient," page 283, for more whole-grain guidance.

Beans. Great sources of protein, fiber, and amino acids, beans are affordable and delicious staples of a diet that promotes total health. Use dried beans and soak them a full twenty-four hours—it makes them more digestible and helps them cook up in less time. This does require some forethought and time, but little extra actual labor. Once the beans have soaked, rinse them, put them in a pot, cover with two inches of water, and toss in a small handful of salt; then simmer over medium-low heat until tender. Cook up a pot on the weekend, and you'll have beans for the week. If you choose canned beans, be sure to check labels for HFCS and other sugars and additives.

Nuts and seeds. Nuts and seeds are a cornerstone of healthy eating, so keep plenty on hand where you can reach them easily. Great choices include walnuts, almonds, pecans, sunflower and pumpkin seeds, flax seeds, and nut butters, including peanut, almond, and cashew butter. But don't go overboard. After buying a bag of nuts and seeds, store half in the freezer and the other half in a see-through airtight container in the pantry, so you'll have some at the ready while maintaining a stash for maximum freshness. While some packaged trail mixes are healthy, beware of those with added sugar and oils.

Healthy oils. Look for cold- or expeller-pressed versions of sunflower oil (for searing and other high-heat uses), extra-virgin olive oil (for baking, roasting, and sautéing), walnut oil (for salad dressings), and toasted sesame oil (for flavoring stir-fries, slaws, and salads after cooking). To keep your oils fresh, buy only as much as you will use in a few months. Buy them in opaque bottles (when available) to protect them from UV damage, and store them in a cool place to avoid damage from heat.

Natural sweeteners. Keeping added sugars to a minimum is a key part of healthy eating. If you like to sweeten your coffee or tea, consider stevia, a plant-based sweetener that's calorie-free but doesn't have the health risks associated with artificial sweeteners. (It's available in crystal or liquid form in most grocery stores.) Local honey, maple syrup, and turbinado sugar (a minimally processed sugar derived from sugarcane) are less processed than white sugar, but don't fool yourself into thinking they're good for you—use them in moderation.

Herbs and spices. These flavor enhancers offer a host of antioxidants and health benefits in addition to adding taste. Keep dried herbs in a dark, cool drawer for up to six months—after that, they begin to lose potency and flavor. Herbs and spices widely hailed for their health benefits include cinnamon (good for regulating blood-sugar levels), turmeric (a powerful anti-inflammatory), cayenne (boosts circulation), ginger (aids digestion), and garlic (has antimicrobial properties). Whatever your favorite spice is, stock it and use it. Flavor helps make the food you cook more satisfying to your taste buds.

Beverages. White and green teas are antioxidant powerhouses that may help with weight loss through a mild metabolic boost. Steep them, ice them, and pour some in your water bottle or travel mug. Those powerful plant compounds are water soluble, so drink up! While they contain a small amount of caffeine (10 to 25 mg on average), they also contain an amino acid called theanine, which has a calming yet focusing effect on our brains. If you don't like the taste (or have yet to acquire a taste for it), consider making a tea concentrate and tossing it in your morning smoothie. Herbal teas are another healthy choice. If you choose to drink wine, choose red for the heart-healthy antioxidants, keeping in mind that "moderation" means up to one glass a day for women, two glasses per day for men. While there's no better beverage than filtered water, if you're weaning yourself off soda or just "don't like the taste" of water, try sparkling water with a splash of antioxidant-rich pomegranate or tart cherry juice (read labels carefully to make sure you're getting 100 percent juice and nothing containing HFCS).

Step 3: Plan and Shop

Planning your meals and arming yourself with a shopping list is a key part of the puzzle. This will provide focus when you're in the store, which, never forget, is set up to sell you the products the grocers most want to move, not to help you find nutritious ingredients. How specific your plan is depends on your personality and comfort level with shopping and cooking.

If you're a planner by nature and you're starting from scratch, try planning out a week's worth of meals and creating your shopping list from there. See pages 280–81 for a shopping list template that can help guide you on what to buy. If you're pretty comfortable in the kitchen and the thought of planning all your meals gives you the shivers, it's not absolutely necessary. Your grocery list can merely focus on restocking your pantry and buying the most appealing fresh ingredients (such as produce and fish) so that you can throw meals together without having to think about them too much.

If you're in the middle somewhere—you don't mind meal planning but don't always have time or the inclination to map out the next seven days—choose one or two dishes and plan to make big batches. Buy the ingredients for those, and use a combination of leftovers and pantry staples to create dishes on the fly for the rest of your meals.

Regardless of your meal-planning approach, it's vital to sit down to make a list before you head to the grocery store. It will make shopping less stressful—no more wondering what you're forgetting while standing at the checkout counter—and make you infinitely more likely to get home with a bevy of good options.

At the grocery store, first things first: make sure you have food in your stomach before you enter the store. If you're hungry while shopping, low blood sugar can compromise your ability to think clearly and make wise decisions, and you'll be much more susceptible to impulse buys.

Once you arrive at the store, shop the produce section first. This is where the majority of your nutrients should come from, so it deserves top priority. You'll also think most clearly at the beginning of your shopping trip, so put that clarity to good use in buying fruits and vegetables. Because produce is seasonal and thus constantly changing, seeing what's available can spark your creativity and make you more excited about the rest of your shopping trip.

Then pick up your lean proteins for the week, such as beans and legumes, seafood, poultry, and meat. After that, it's just a matter of restocking the pantry items that you've noted on your list, and choosing *not* to buy the unhealthy foods you just can't resist. You can skip some aisles altogether.

Step 4: Revamp the Kitchen

Now that you've cleared out the junk and stocked up on healthy food, optimize your storage spaces to make getting to the good stuff convenient and easy.

Refrigerator

- **Shelves.** Think top to bottom. Just as store owners boost sales of certain items by placing them at eye level, you can capitalize on the most visible portion of your fridge by storing healthy grab-and-go items in clear containers on the **top** shelf, like precut fruit and veggies and leftovers that need to be eaten soon. Healthy drink options go here, too, such as filtered or bubbly water, and maybe a 100-percent fruit juice for a splash of flavor added to the bubbly. Less perishable staples can go on the **middle** shelf: nut butters and nuts, yogurt, and whole-grain breads. Reserve the **bottom** shelf for bulk items, such as cooked grains or beans, and for anything you

Shopping List Template

So that you always have the makings of a healthy meal on hand, include foods from the following categories on each grocery store run. This is just a sampling within each category, but it will give you a good idea of what to shop for.

Fruits and vegetables

Eat with the seasons as much as possible, and supplement with frozen versions when supply is limited. Check the Environmental Working Group's list of the Dirty Dozen to learn which twelve fruits and vegetables are the most pesticide-laden so you can opt for organic on those items, or focus on the Clean 15—the least contaminated varieties of produce. The lists change periodically; look for the latest at http://www.ewg.org/foodnews/.

High-quality animal protein and sources of plant protein (keep two or three on hand)

- Wild seafood (versus farm-raised)
- Organic grass-fed sources of meat, eggs, and dairy
- Organic, non-GMO soy (edamame, tempeh, miso, and tofu)
- Beans
- Protein powder for smoothies (whey, soy, brown rice, hemp, pea)

Fiber-rich whole grains (keep at least two or three on hand)

• Brown rice	• Millet	• Steel-cut oatmeal
• Quinoa	• Barley	

Nuts, seeds, and nut butters (keep at least two on hand)

• Walnuts	• Almond butter	• Pumpkin seeds
• Almonds	• Cashew butter	• Flaxseed
• Pecans	• Organic peanut butter	• Sesame seeds
• Cashews	• Coconut "butter"	• Chia seeds

Healthy oils and fats
(keep extra-virgin olive oil and at least one more on hand)

- Extra-virgin olive oil
- Coconut oil
- Sesame oil
- Walnut oil
- Flaxseed oil
- Avocado oil
- Grapeseed oil
- Ghee (clarified butter)

Probiotic foods (keep one or two on hand)

- Organic Greek yogurt (unsweetened)
- Kefir
- Miso
- Kimchee
- Tempeh
- Traditionally made sauerkraut
- Sourdough bread made with sourdough starter (not commercial yeast)

Beverages

- Green tea
- White tea
- Herbal teas
- Seltzer water
- 100-percent fruit juice (for diluting in seltzer water to make a healthy soda replacement)
- Organic milk (or almond milk, soy milk, or coconut milk)
- Tart cherry juice
- Pomegranate juice

Desserts

- Dark chocolate (ideally, at least 72 percent cocoa and organic)
- Dried fruit (unsweetened)
- Fresh fruit
- Frozen berries/cherries

don't want a visual reminder of every time you open the fridge, such as that leftover birthday cake.

- **Crisper drawers.** Keep it simple: dedicate one drawer for fruits, the other for veggies. This also helps keep veggies fresher longer, since they won't be exposed to the methylene gas emitted by fruit as it ripens.

- **The door.** Again, think top to bottom for your condiments. Healthiest options like salsa, mustards, and fruit spreads go in the most visible, most easily accessible spaces, while oily, salty, or sugary condiments—mayonnaise, soy sauce, barbecue sauce, ketchup—go lower down.

- **The freezer.** Keeping it simple will help keep things organized—we've all faced the crazy jumble of a disorganized freezer (and quickly shut the door on it). One shelf can be for frozen fruits and vegetables, another for meats and extra portions of previous meals. Items that keep longer in the freezer, such as flaxseed and whole-grain flours, are easily stored in the door.

Pantry

The same principle applies to your cupboards: Give your most convenient healthy options a place of prominence. Put your staples—such as grains, dried beans, and canned tuna and salmon—at eye level. Then store your healthy snacks—such as dried fruit, nuts, and roasted edamame—and your herbs, teas, salt, and pepper on the other shelves. And if you've got anything on hand that doesn't fit into your plan of eating for total health, store it in an opaque container on a high shelf—you'll be less likely to reach for it if you can't see it.

Eat Like an Ancient

Minimizing refined-grain products like conventional pasta and white rice is key to your kitchen makeover, but that doesn't mean you're stuck eating brown rice night after night. Grains such as spelt, buckwheat, quinoa, millet, barley, and amaranth have been cultivated and eaten by humans for millennia, and they remain an excellent source of nutrition. Millet has a crunch that makes a great addition to granola or muesli; barley has a chewiness that makes it a hearty addition to chunky soups or the start of a salad; quinoa has a nuttiness that makes it an appealing alternative to rice.

Consumed in their whole, unprocessed state, these grains are excellent sources of slow-burning carbohydrates—so-called because their fiber content means they take longer to digest than simple carbs, which include refined grains and sugars. As a result, we feel full longer and we don't experience the fluctuations in blood-sugar and insulin levels that can dramatically undermine our energy levels, mood, and brain function—and ultimately our health. Slow-burning carbs are also beneficial because they increase brain levels of the mood-regulating hormone serotonin.

These grains are typically available in whole form, although some are also ground into flour. Most cook up in a pot with water—toasting beforehand intensifies their flavor but isn't necessary. Try using them in place of pasta or rice, tossing them into soups, or as a base for chili, curries, and stews. They are becoming increasingly easy to find in mainstream grocery stores, and even in big-box stores. Look for them in the rice aisle or near the dried beans. They are also more and more commonly used to make pastas, breads, pretzels, and baking mixes. These products may be in the "health food" section of your grocery store, or they may appear alongside more conventional alternatives.

Another important benefit of ancient grains is that many of them do not contain gluten—a protein that's a major component of wheat, barley, and rye and may be present in some oat products due to cross-contamination in the food-supply chain. Because we eat so much wheat and so many wheat products, many people are developing sensitivities to gluten, which can result in indigestion, gas, bloating, joint pain, brain fog, and weight gain, among other problems. For those who have a true allergy to gluten—a condition known as celiac disease—eating wheat can trigger an autoimmune response and lead to serious consequences. Even if you don't have any issues with gluten, it's beneficial to add gluten-free grains to your repertoire so that you become less likely to develop a sensitivity to it in the future, and as always we are looking to increase the variety of foods we eat to maximize their benefits. Many of our clients who make an effort to eat less gluten report shedding a few pounds as a result.

Eating Pitfalls and Solutions

What recurring scenarios trip you up the most when it comes to eating well? Take some time to really think through what triggers your worst eating episodes. We have found that people who plan in advance and keep healthier options on hand often avoid the pitfalls and temptations that can sabotage their goals. This planning occurs at home, then at the grocery store, and then in the way you store your foods. See the chart below for some tips on how to avoid common traps.

Common Challenge	Antidote
Skipping breakfast	Buy or make individual serving-sized packages of nuts that, along with easily portable fruit—such as an apple, pear, orange, or banana—you can grab for breakfast on your way out the door and eat en route or at your desk. Although we discourage "grab and go" as a regular habit, it is healthier than other options.
Getting hungry before lunch—and resorting to the vending machine	Pack a healthy snack *every day*—such as Greek yogurt and fruit, hummus and carrots, whole-grain crackers and low-fat cheese, nuts, or nut butters. Think of options that combine whole-food carbs, protein, and healthy fat.
Reaching for coffee or sugary snacks in the afternoon to ward off low blood sugar	Take a ten-minute walk around the block or the office first, then reach for a healthy carbohydrate paired with protein, such as dried fruit and nuts. Also try green tea.
Snacking while waiting for dinner	Hold off on alcoholic beverages until dinner is in front of you—drinking on an empty stomach has been shown to increase premeal snacking. Drink a glass of water, which will ease that empty-stomach feeling. And if you must have a snack, make it vegetables, such as raw carrots, sliced zucchini, or strips of red bell pepper. After dinner, prepare a snack to have at the ready for the next night.

Common Challenge	Antidote
Eating before bed	Brush your teeth right after dinner—it can help dissuade you from putting anything other than water in your mouth. If your late-night eating is of the mindless variety, find something else to do with your hands—knitting, prepping vegetables for your next cooking session, or reading a book. If you're truly hungry, go ahead and eat a snack that provides some healthy fat as well as some slow-burning carbs, such as a brown rice cake with peanut butter, a sliver of avocado and low-fat cottage cheese, or an apple with almond butter.

Meal Planning

Once you've "detoxed" your fridge and pantry and then restocked them with the essential ingredients for healthy eating, you're ready to start following a weekly meal plan. For most people, knowing when and what they're going to eat can curb overeating. For instance, if you know that you have all the ingredients for a ten-minute meal at home, you won't feel the need to scarf down pretzels on your drive home. Being prepared reduces that urgent "I need food now!" feeling. And yet being too rigid with your menu can backfire. In our practice, we teach the idea of structured flexibility—using a weekly meal plan as a guide, but one that you can adjust based on the time, energy, and ingredients you have on hand.

Before you sit down to write a meal plan, you need to know what constitutes a meal. For optimal blood-sugar balance and overall health, remember the "magic formula" you learned about in chapter 10: slow-burning carbs from vegetables, fruits, and/or whole grains; lean protein;

and healthy fat. Eating this way helps stabilize blood-sugar and insulin levels, which means fewer mood swings, fewer cravings and bouts of over-eating, a lower risk of diabetes and most chronic illnesses, as well as sustained mental and physical energy. The formula holds true for snacks, too.

Balanced Snacks

Slow-Burning Carbohydrate	Lean Protein	Healthy Fat	Extras
Example 1: Brown rice cracker	1 whole egg	⅛ avocado	Garlic, cracked pepper, drizzle of balsamic vinegar
Example 2: Tomato slices	Hummus	Drizzle of extra-virgin olive oil	

Step One: In a typical week, you'll spend fifteen minutes thinking about what you'll eat in the next seven days—maybe it's on Sunday evening, or on one relatively quiet weekday morning, or even at your desk while you're waiting for a conference call to start. That way, you'll have to shop only once during the week, buying everything you'll need to make the meals you've already planned. Occasionally, you'll want to try out a new recipe that requires a special ingredient, or you'll decide to try experimenting with a new grain. But mostly, you won't need to buy special ingredients—you'll simply restock your pantry and pick up a healthy assortment of fruits and vegetables that will change throughout the year depending on the season.

Step Two: Find the times of the week when it's convenient for you to do the majority of your cooking—you can chop several onions or cloves of garlic at once, for example, and store what you don't use in that instance in the fridge or freezer, dramatically reducing the prep time and cleanup for a weeknight stir-fry. It's also helpful to cook several batches of healthy basics over the weekend, including one protein (such as beans), one grain (such as quinoa), and one vegetable (such as grilled peppers in the summer or roasted squash in the winter—or a favorite combination of mixed roasted vegetables anytime). You can serve the three together for dinner on the weekend. Then, on Monday you can add the vegetables to the sandwich you pack for lunch and use the beans in a simple quesadilla with a side of sliced tomatoes for dinner. The quinoa can serve as a bed for over-easy eggs for Tuesday's breakfast, and you can transform the remaining beans into a main-dish salad with a simple vinaigrette dressing and the addition of crumbled feta and fresh herbs. Wednesday you'll need to cook again—make a double batch of steel-cut oatmeal and save the leftovers for another breakfast. Cook a soup that night and serve it over the remaining quinoa to make it a filling meal. Those leftovers make a great lunch for Thursday, and the last of the beans pairs nicely with a simple green salad and whole-grain tortillas with avocado for dinner that night.

If this sounds too ambitious, start slowly. Pick one new dinner recipe to try each week. Or start with breakfast—try something new, and if you like it, keep it for your repertoire.

Better Brown Bagging

Many clients report that planning healthy lunches is especially tricky. These strategies can help.

- Plan your lunches for the week ahead of time.
- Keep last-minute items on hand: canned tuna, salmon, nut butters, brown rice tortillas, whole-grain crackers, hummus.
- Pack condiments separately to prevent lunches from getting soggy.
- Grill or roast veggies to use all week—add to sandwiches and wraps or pair with cheese for a tasty and filling snack.
- Invest in a mini cooler to keep food fresh.
- Freeze drinks overnight, then place them in the cooler to keep your lunch cool (it will thaw by lunchtime).

Mix-and-Match Meals

The charts below will help you create nutritious, creative meals that contain a combination of slow-burning carbohydrates, lean protein, and healthy fat. Use them as a guide and an inspiration for meal planning—or creating meals spontaneously out of what you have in your refrigerator and pantry.

For each meal or snack, you'll pick food(s) from the carbohydrate columns (vegetables, fruits, and/or whole grains), food(s) from the protein column, and food(s) from the healthy fats column. As you'll see, nuts and nut butters appear in both the protein and fats columns, because they are good sources of both nutrients.

While the charts are broken into breakfast, lunch, and dinner, you'll see many of the same foods in all three charts. Think outside the box! If you love traditional breakfast foods, have them for dinner. Incorporate dinner leftovers into your breakfast. Moving away from certain foods for certain meals—especially a pattern of eating only baked goods and cereal for breakfast—will help you follow the principles outlined in chapter 10. Including multiple servings of vegetables and/or fruits (in the carbohydrate category) with every meal will help you build your plant base, and the add-ons at the bottom of each chart will not only enhance flavor, they'll add to your intake of antioxidants and other beneficial phytochemicals. Think of them as bonus points.

Note the total daily servings you're aiming for in each category (listed at the top of each column) and the serving sizes for various foods (listed below the charts), but keep in mind that these are estimates only; people's individual recommendations will vary. The focus here is on eating balanced meals.

Breakfast

Slow-Burning Carbohydrate		Lean Protein	Healthy Fat
Vegetable/Fruit *9–11 servings/day*	**Whole Grain** *2–4 servings/day*	*6–9 servings/day*	*9–11 servings/day*
Fresh or frozen berries (blueberries, raspberries, strawberries) Tart cherries Apricots Apples Prunes Banana Orange Grapefruit Sweet potatoes Peppers (all) Broccoli Kale Spinach Mushrooms Squash Bok choy Tomatoes Onion	Brown rice tortilla Corn tortilla Oatmeal Steel-cut oats Five-grain hot cereal Whole-grain porridge or cereal (use barley, teff, buckwheat, farro, or amaranth) Muesli Whole-grain English muffin Whole-grain waffle Whole-grain pancake	Nuts (almonds, walnuts, pistachios, pecans, pine nuts) Nut butter (almond, cashew, walnut, organic peanut butter) Eggs (organic and omega-3 fortified) Non-GMO/organic soy milk Organic Greek yogurt Organic kefir Organic cottage cheese Organic milk Smoked salmon Sardines Protein powder (whey, brown rice, pea, hemp)	Flaxseed (ground) Hemp seeds Chia seeds Nut/seed butter (almond butter, cashew butter, walnut butter, organic peanut butter, sunflower seed butter) Nuts (almonds, cashews, walnuts, pistachios, pecans, pine nuts) Avocado Extra-virgin olive oil Canola oil Avocado oil Coconut oil Pesto
Healthy Add-ons	Organic cocoa powder Cinnamon Nutmeg Turmeric	Cumin Ginger Parsley Rosemary Garlic	Oregano Thyme Sage Black pepper Basil

Lunch

Slow-Burning Carbohydrate		Lean Protein	Healthy Fat
Vegetable/Fruit *9–11 servings/day*	**Whole Grain** *2–4 servings/day*	*6–9 servings/day*	*9–11 servings/day*
Spinach	Quinoa	Beans (black, pinto, cannellini)	Nuts
Bok choy	Brown rice	Lentils	Nut/seed butter
Mixed greens	Black rice	Chickpeas	Ground flax-seed
Swiss chard	Barley	Hummus	Hemp seeds
Celery	Millet	Non-GMO soybeans/edamame	Chia seeds
Onion	Teff		Pumpkin seeds
Peppers (all)	Farro	Black bean burger	Sunflower seeds
Tomatoes	Brown rice tortilla	Wild fish	Extra-virgin olive oil
Brussels sprouts	Corn tortilla	Lean, grass-fed beef and bison	Grapeseed oil
Cabbage	Whole-grain tortilla	Poultry	Avocado oil
Beets	Sprouted whole-grain bread	Pork	Coconut oil
Artichoke	Whole-grain pita	Turkey burger	Canola oil
Cauliflower	Brown rice pasta	(Choose organic meat when possible.)	Pesto
Broccoli	Quinoa pasta		Tahini
Sweet potatoes	Whole-wheat pasta	Canned salmon	Avocado
Squash		Nuts	
Carrots		Organic Greek yogurt	
Berries			
Apple			
Pear			
Tart cherries			
Papaya			
Healthy Add-ons	Turmeric Cumin Ginger Parsley Basil	Rosemary Oregano Thyme Sage Cilantro	Black pepper Organic cocoa powder Cinnamon Nutmeg

Dinner

Slow-Burning Carbohydrate		Lean Protein	Healthy Fat
Vegetable/Fruit *9–11 servings/day*	**Whole Grain** *2–4 servings/day*	*6–9 servings/day*	*9–11 servings/day*
Kale Spinach Collards Bok choy Mixed greens Swiss chard Mushrooms Celery Onion Zucchini Tomatoes Brussels sprouts Beets Carrots Sweet potatoes Squash Artichoke Cauliflower Broccoli Berries Apple Mango	Quinoa Brown rice Black rice Barley Millet Teff Whole-grain tortilla Brown rice tortilla Corn tortilla Whole-grain pita Sprouted whole-grain bread Brown rice pasta Quinoa pasta Whole-grain pasta	Beans Lentils Black bean burger Bean soups Chickpeas Non-GMO minimally processed soy (edamame, tempeh, miso) Non-GMO tofu Wild fish Lean, grass-fed beef, bison Poultry Pork Turkey burger Protein powder Canned salmon Sardines Organic Greek yogurt	Nut/seed butter Nuts Ground flaxseed Hemp seeds Chia seeds Sunflower seeds Pumpkin seeds Pesto Tahini Avocado Extra-virgin olive oil Grapeseed oil Avocado oil Coconut oil Organic ghee (clarified butter) Walnut oil
Healthy Add-ons	Turmeric Cumin Ginger Parsley Basil	Rosemary Oregano Thyme Sage Cilantro	Black pepper Organic cocoa powder Cinnamon Nutmeg

Sample breakfasts

- Green smoothie with baby kale and spinach, mixed berries, whey protein powder, banana, ground flaxseed, and cooled green tea
- Whole-grain tortilla with scrambled omega-3-fortified eggs, spinach, roasted vegetables (left over from dinner), and pesto
- Oatmeal with dried tart cherries, chopped nuts, and ground flaxseed
- Mixed-grain pancake with mixed berries, protein powder, and coconut milk

Sample lunches

- Brown rice tortilla with baby spinach, chopped sweet potato, black beans, roasted chicken, avocado, and salsa; papaya with lime juice
- Black bean chili; steamed broccoli, carrots, and corn; cashews
- Mixed greens salad with farro, roasted chicken, sunflower seeds, pistachios, and balsamic vinaigrette; blueberries
- Whole-grain pita, turkey burger, shredded slaw (purple cabbage and carrot), pesto; apple

Sample dinners

- Mixed ancient grains, wild salmon with mango chutney, roasted Brussels sprouts, fennel salad
- Spinach salad with strawberries, red onion, and pine nuts; dressing with extra-virgin olive oil; egg frittata with onion, broccolini, and fresh parsley
- Lentil soup, roasted cauliflower, kale salad with pine nuts and walnut-oil vinaigrette
- Shrimp kabob with tomato and zucchini, quinoa pasta with walnut pesto

Serving Sizes

This chart shows serving sizes (as opposed to portions). Keep your total daily servings for each category in mind, noted in the charts above.

Foods	Serving Size
CARBOHYDRATES (Grains)	½ cup cooked cereal ¾ cup cold cereal ⅓ cup cooked grains 1 slice bread ⅓ cup cooked pasta
CARBOHYDRATES (Vegetables & Fruit)	½ cup cooked vegetables 1 cup raw vegetables 1 cup berries ¼ cup dried fruit 1 small piece of fruit
PROTEIN	1 oz. meat 1 oz. seafood 1 oz. fish 7 g protein powder ½ cup cooked beans, peas, or lentils 1 oz. cheese 8 oz. milk 2 tbsp. nut butter
FATS	⅛ avocado 1 tsp. extra-virgin olive oil 1 tbsp. pesto 2 tbsp. ground flaxseed, chia seeds, or hemp seeds ¼ oz. nuts 1 tsp. butter 2 tsp. nut butter

Grocery Store Time-Savers

Food items that make weeknight cooking a snap:

- Skinless, boneless chicken
- Canned beans (to avoid the BPA in the can lining, look for beans in Tetra Paks)
- Grated or shredded cheese
- Sliced lean meats
- Chopped, sliced, prewashed produce
- Chopped nuts
- Frozen vegetables
- Pre-cooked grains

Healthy Cooking 101

Now it's time to get cooking. Here are a few techniques you'll use again and again. Play with them all, master one or two, and you'll always be no more than a few minutes away from a healthy meal.

Steaming. Okay, steamed vegetables don't make many people's mouth water. But here's the beauty of steaming—it's really simple, and it preserves the nutrients in food better than any other method of cooking. Once your veggies are steamed, you can add a drizzle of olive oil and get the flavor boost fat provides with a fraction of the calories it takes to cook with fat in most other methods. All you need is a large pot with a lid and a steamer insert. With those basic pieces of equipment, you can prepare any vegetable in minutes: put a small amount of water in the bottom of the pot, place the steamer insert inside, then put your chopped veggies on the steam tray. Place the lid on top and turn the heat up to medium. Veggies are done when their color is most intense and they are fork-tender. For time-crunched evenings, use the microwave. Pour a little water in a Pyrex dish and cover the dish with a BPA-free silicone cover, leaving a slight opening for the steam to release.

Stir-frying. Quick, easy, and efficient, stir-frying sears food over high heat so that it's the perfect combination of crispy and tender. You'll need a large pan, a small amount of high-heat-tolerant oil (such as grapeseed, peanut, or avocado), and a combination of meat, seafood, or tofu and vegetables that are cut into uniformly sized pieces. Heat the pan over high heat, using just enough oil to coat the pan. When a drop of water sizzles and immediately evaporates, the pan is ready. Add the food item that takes the longest to cook (such as broccoli), stir it constantly for a minute or two, then keep adding ingredients in order of their cooking time, adding the fastest-cooking ingredient last (such as shrimp). Drizzle with a little soy sauce and/or lemon juice just before turning off the heat, and *voilà*! Dinner.

Slow-cooking. Imagine throwing some ingredients in a magical contraption in the morning, flipping a switch before leaving the house, then returning home after work to find an entire dinner waiting for you, ready to eat. With a slow cooker (otherwise known by the brand name Crock-Pot), this dream comes true. Perfect for soups, stews, chilis, slow-cooked meats and veggies, and much more, a slow cooker does all the fussing for you—no watching the clock or worrying about overcooking. Invest in a slow-cooker cookbook or find recipes online.

Roasting. The same method we have been using to cook meats and seafood can be applied to cooking vegetables. In fact, we'd be hard-pressed to think of a vegetable that doesn't taste better when roasted. Squash, parsnips, sweet potatoes, zucchini, peppers, eggplant, garlic, cauliflower, and even the often-maligned Brussels sprouts are transformed during roasting. Greens such as kale and collards crisp up into tasty chips, and beets and cauliflower develop a caramelized layer to bring out their natural sweetness. The basic rule of thumb is to chop your veggie into same-sized pieces, toss it in a little olive oil, and season with salt and pepper. Place on a rimmed baking sheet in a 350°F oven. Stir occasionally and remove when the edges begin to brown. You do have to get comfortable with chopping—and keep an eye on things so the brown edges don't tip over into charred territory. Otherwise, this cooking method is basically foolproof.

Exercise: Mindful Cooking

Because cooking is a sensory experience, it provides lots of opportunities for mindfulness. Pick an instance when you have sufficient time and quiet to focus in the kitchen; avoid multitasking, such as talking on the phone or with your spouse or children as you cook. As you're prepping, focus on the feel of your hands on the knife as you chop garlic or vegetables. Absorb the sound the blade makes as it cuts through the food and hits the cutting board. Notice how the aroma affects your nose, and what chain reaction it may cause in your body—your mouth may start watering, or your body may want to retreat from the odor if it's pungent. While you're focused on the physical sensations of cooking, take note of what's happening in your mind. Are you noticing anticipation or excitement about the food? Are you feeling proud of taking care of yourself? Are there any insights bubbling up to the surface of your awareness?

Your "New Normal" Kitchen Routine

For most of us, it's important to continue to keep in mind that not every meal has to be an event. Occasionally, you'll prepare something quickly to eat on the run—but with proper planning and mindful awareness, you can make even quick meals and snacks healthy. Other times, you can make preparing and eating your food a lovely, nurturing opportunity to get your mind and body back in sync. How much time you spend on each meal and snack will vary based on your schedule, your preference, and your willingness to slow down. The important thing is to shift away from ingrained habits of mindless eating and toward consciously choosing food that promotes your health and builds vital energy. How much better you feel will be its own reward and give you motivation to continue.

As you're preparing your food, invite all your senses to the table. Experience the feel, smell, sight, and sound of the food as it cooks. Focusing in this way may inspire you to pull out your favorite dishes, light candles, bring in some flowers, put a sprig of parsley on the plate just to pretty it up, or enjoy a leisurely whiff of your food before you bite into it. You'll be less likely to dine and dash and will be able to sit and truly savor each bite.

Insights and Inspirations: Marsha, age 47

Growing up, it seemed like my mom was always in the kitchen— cooking, washing dishes, sweeping, talking on the phone. She joked that she wasn't allowed out of the room. When I became an adult, I prided myself on NOT cooking—I didn't want to be a prisoner in my own kitchen like my mom. The prepared foods in the deli case were my best friends. But then I found out I had high blood pressure and cholesterol, and I had to be more careful about what I ate. Despite everything I thought I knew about cooking—how it was drudgery and took up all your time—I found out I loved being in the kitchen. I love that you make a big mess, use your hands, think creatively, and then usually have something tasty to eat when you're done. Sometimes I do think cooking is a pain, but by the time I get into the rhythm of chopping and stirring, I realize I'm having fun. I'd still like a robot to come in and do all the dishes, but I don't miss microwaved meals. At all. And I can do anything—even dishes—to a good soundtrack!

An Attitude of Gratitude

To elevate the act of cooking from a chore into something uplifting and inspiring, try incorporating a gratitude practice into your meal. **A regular practice of focusing on thankful feelings has been shown repeatedly to have a host of health benefits, including a stronger immune**

system, lower blood pressure, and a greater sense of connection to others. In our practice, we've seen firsthand the shift that happens when people spend a few moments expressing gratitude: it transforms a snack or a meal from simply a time to refuel to an opportunity to connect with the web of life. It encourages us to slow down and savor our food and invites mindfulness to have a spot at the table. Not only is it a spiritual and health-promoting practice, but there is even a physiological rationale for "giving thanks" before a meal. The practice allows for a shift in the body as it prepares for the approaching food. Our attention is focused on the meal—our mouths begin to salivate, releasing the first of many enzymes necessary to properly digest our foods. Our bodies make a switch from the sympathetic nervous system, which has kept us revved up all day to deal with stressors, to the parasympathetic nervous system, which calms us and allows for better digestion.

Your gratitude practice needn't be formal. Here are a few ways to up your gratitude quotient, particularly around eating:

- Offer grace or a prayer from your own spiritual tradition—out loud or silently—before digging in. Varying the words will increase your attentiveness to the practice.

- Imagine each person and animal involved in getting the food from the field or farm to your table, and thank them for their efforts. Consider all it took to create these nutrients to take care of your body.

- Think of three things you're thankful for—they can be from any area of your life (not just regarding the food you're about to eat). The more specific, the better. For example, instead of saying you're thankful for your husband (in general), you could give thanks for "the way my husband touched my back this morning when he asked how I slept." Either list them mentally, share them with your eating partners, or write them down in a notebook.

- Take turns going around the table and sharing one thing you're thankful for, or thanking one person involved in growing, delivering, selling, or preparing the food.

Mind over Menu

Now that we've established that preparing your own food is a fundamental piece of healthy eating, let's talk about eating outside the home. Restaurants are, after all, an integral part of modern life. In fact, 47 percent of all the money spent on food in America is spent in restaurants. Even when you're cooking most of your own food, you'll end up having a lunch out here and a dinner out there—more if you travel for work or for play.

We're happy to say that it is absolutely possible to eat healthfully when dining out. But it's not easy. And here's the number-one reason why: typical restaurant meals average about 1,120 calories. That's as much as what some people should consume in an entire day! Besides the extra calories, restaurant food is rife with health-harming fats and refined sugars and grains. Like grocery stores, restaurants are businesses whose aim is to sell you food. It's no accident that your server asks, "Would you like one of our signature cocktails?" or "Who's ready for dessert?" The mere power of suggestion makes it more likely that you will overindulge—which is great for a restaurant's bottom line but hazardous to your well-being.

A lot of psychological components play into our eating-out habits. Even though we are eating at restaurants more often than ever before, we still think of eating out as a splurge-worthy occasion. Sure, if you eat out only once every few months, you *could* enjoy an appetizer, multiple drinks, an entrée, and dessert without it having a negative lasting effect on your health. But when you're going out to eat once a week or more, those extra calories add up quickly. Moreover, eating for total health means redefining your concept of reward. Tuning in to your true needs in the moment will help you find rewards that genuinely support your health.

Keep in mind that even if you head into a restaurant with the best of intentions, if your dining partner opts to splurge on a cheeseburger with fries, you become much more likely to do the same.

The key to keeping your wits about you when eating out is to *have a strategy before you go in.* Look at the menu online before going to the restaurant and make a plan about what you will order—or at least consider options. Also spend a few minutes sitting quietly, envisioning the occasion. Visualize yourself choosing food that sounds appealing and refreshingly healthy. Let yourself feel how good it will feel to walk out of the restaurant without being overstuffed and bloated. Remember that you are being mindful of your food choices because you want and deserve to feel radiantly healthy and energetic. Think about what you'll say when the server comes over to your table (see the chart below for ideas). Before you open your eyes, choose where you want to place your focus when you're at the restaurant—on the company you'll be with, or the pretty surroundings, or the fact that someone else is preparing and cleaning up after your meal while you relax. Later, when you're at the restaurant, take a deep breath and remember the images that came up for you during this visualization to help you stick to your plan.

When your host/server says:	Answer:
"Can I start you off with a drink?"	"Water would be great, thanks." "I'll wait until I decide what I'm having for dinner."
"Would you like some bread and butter (or chips and salsa, or breadsticks and hummus) to get you started?"	"No thanks, I'm holding out for the soup/salad/entrée." Pass the basket to the far end of the table or ask the server to remove it.
"What would you like for an appetizer?"	"I'll have the soup (or salad)." "Nothing, thanks."
"And for your entrée?"	"We'd like to split the _____." "Please bring me half the entrée and wrap the other half for me to take home."

| "Can I bring you another drink?" | "No thanks, I'm going to switch to water." |
| "Who has room for dessert?" | "Not me! I'm just right. Dinner was delicious." |

While you're reading the menu, look for terms that hint at how the food was prepared and how much fat it contains. While we advocate consuming healthy fat, most fats used in restaurants are the unhealthy kind—including trans fats and omega-6-rich vegetable oils. Restaurants use these fats with a heavy hand to make the food more flavorful, which results in a calorie total that's sky high.

Low-fat preparation	High-fat preparation
Baked or broiled	Breaded or fried
Stir-fried	Alfredo/mystery sauce
Poached	Au gratin/smothered
Grilled	Escalloped
Roasted	Flaky (as in pie crust)
Boiled or steamed	Parmigiano

Beyond being a savvy menu reader, you have another invaluable skill when it comes to getting a healthy meal in a restaurant: your voice. You have every right to ask for what you need and to have your requests honored. You also are well within your bounds to ask about how certain dishes are prepared, to ask for substitutions (such as a baked potato or green salad instead of fries), and to have sauces and dressings served on the side. Be polite, but don't be shy.

And finally, consider using eating-out experiences to try something new—something you're unlikely to make at home. Go to the new vegan restaurant in town, or try a new type of seafood. Who knows—you may find a new favorite dish to try at home.

Drinking and Dining

We can't talk about staying healthy while eating out without talking about alcohol. Beer, wine, and cocktails are all hefty sources of calories in their own right (see "Calorie Counts for Common Drinks" for more details), and drinking while dining makes you more likely to choose unhealthy foods and to eat more overall. Research has shown that people given alcohol before or during a meal ate more than those who didn't consume alcohol. Ask yourself—do I really need a drink to enjoy myself at a restaurant? If you do decide to imbibe, the simplest way to cut back on alcohol is to drink a full glass of water before and after any alcoholic drink. And try asking your server to bring the drink with food, since eating while drinking will help you avoid tipsiness and the desire to throw caution to the wind and order the nachos.

Calorie Counts for Common Drinks

While *serving sizes* are listed here, the *portion* you're served may be significantly larger—and therefore more caloric (not to mention more alcoholic).

Red wine	(5 oz.)	125
White wine	(5 oz.)	121
Champagne	(4 oz.)	86
Regular beer	(12 oz.)	153
Light beer	(12 oz.)	103
Bloody Mary	(5 oz.)	120
Cosmopolitan	(2.75 oz.)	146
Mojito	(6 oz.)	170
Piña colada	(9 oz.)	490
Dry martini	(2.25 oz.)	139
Vodka or gin and tonic	(7 oz.)	200
Margarita	(8 oz.)	280

Staying Mindful in a Social Setting

Tuning in to the myriad smells, sights, and feelings of connection to your fellow diners, and to the slowly savored tastes of your food, can help you circumvent many triggers for mindless eating. Other ways to help you stay mindful include putting your fork down after each bite, eating with your nondominant hand, and taking a deep breath between bites—all techniques that help you slow down and think before you bring another bite to your lips. They let your brain catch up to your hands, so you can register that you're satisfied before you end up overeating. Being out at a bustling restaurant or party is stimulating; there's a lot to watch, look at, and hear, which makes it easy to get distracted or overstimulated. There's also often a level of social anxiety, which makes us apt to eat and drink more.

Your mindfulness skills can help you stay centered. Here's a technique to help yourself feel grounded in your body when you're sitting at the table: Bring the soles of both feet to the floor. See if you can feel each one of your ten toes. The simple shift in focus helps you stay present and forces a shift in brain activity from emotional reactivity into a calmer space with greater access to logic and remembering your true needs. And inviting yourself to feel your connection to the ground brings a sense of stability. It also works when you're standing up. Instead of standing with most of your weight on one leg or the other, decide to bring your weight evenly onto both feet. Feel your legs connected to the floor and your spine, torso, neck, and head rising effortlessly out of that solid base.

As you're enjoying the meal, notice how it feels to be consciously choosing to eat healthfully, instead of eating too much too quickly to the point of discomfort, which is the typical pattern at restaurants. Let the feelings of empowerment you notice serve as positive reinforcement for yourself—you *can* make healthy choices, and *this* is what it feels like when you do.

Conclusion:
Making Change Last

At the end of our programs at Duke Integrative Medicine, participants are sometimes hit with apprehension. *Will this approach really be different from the others I've tried? What's this going to mean for my day-to-day life? Will I stick with the practices when things get stressful? Is lasting change really possible?*

Integrating behavior changes into our lives—with the people in our lives—is not always a smooth process. It's important to acknowledge that making changes to your eating habits, even small ones, is a big deal, not only because of the internal work it requires but also because it often means rocking the boat. Eating based on your internal signals instead of the clock, eating slowly, shifting to a plant-based diet—every one of these health-promoting changes means going against the grain of our society's eating culture and perhaps against your own social culture as well.

Practicing mindful eating will often mean being different—in your home, at work, and at a restaurant. It might mean saying no to the chocolate cream pie that your aunt made because it's always been your favorite, or asking for a sliver instead of the big slice she just served you. It might mean bringing your own lunch to an all-day work conference when all your coworkers choose pizza, or asking for sparkling water instead of wine at a party. It might mean asking a waiter for something that's not on the menu at a restaurant, like steamed or roasted vegetables. On a given occasion, you might decide to go with the flow or follow the path of least resistance. Guidelines (as opposed to rules) allow for that.

But you'll find that if you "bend" your guidelines every time it's easier to do so, you'll be bending them all the time. Better to prepare yourself for the discomfort of taking a stand and doing something different.

The more you practice your new skills and habits out in the world, the easier and more comfortable they become, whether you're asking for dressing on the side, taking a deep breath before your next bite, going for a brisk after-dinner walk, or serving meals centered around vegetables. Whatever your changes are, they will slowly but surely become what you do and, after you've been practicing for a long time, part of who you are. In chapter 3 we talked about creating your own food culture. That takes time, but it will begin to feel natural, and it will be strong enough to withstand challenges. You might even find that your changes inspire people around you to make healthy changes of their own.

Regardless of your external environment—supportive and healthy, full of temptation and triggers, or even hostile—the foundation you've built will always be there for you. The mindfulness principles you've been practicing—awareness of the present moment, compassion, and non-judgment—are qualities you can always come back to. They're your home base, and as you continue to cultivate them with daily meditation and the other mindfulness tools you've learned (20 Breaths, Body Scan, the Hunger-Fullness Scan, Loving-Kindness Meditation), the more connected you'll be to your Inner Compass and your values.

Remember, though, that there's no wagon to fall off or competition to fail. As in meditation itself, when your mind wanders off and you bring it back gently to the breath, your habits and your practice may seem to wander off during a stressful or busy time. Unhealthy foods might make their way into your freezer or desk drawer. You might stop your regular morning run. When these kinds of setbacks happen, just notice what's happening—or what happened—and start tuning back in to your mind and your body, and all of the information and wisdom they hold. That compassionate connection to yourself is your most powerful tool.

You've learned a lot about what types of foods lead your body *away* from obesity and chronic illness and toward health—and how powerful your choices are. Choices include shopping on the perimeter of the grocery store, with its abundant vegetables, fruits, and other whole foods (instead of the interior aisles jammed with boxes of processed "ingredients"), or committing to a weekly tennis match with your best friend, or clearing your schedule on Sunday afternoons to make big batches of soups and stews to freeze. Even seemingly small choices, like saying "no thanks" to chips and salsa when you're out, or eating a single cookie instead of three, are powerful. Remember, every bite matters, down to your DNA. Even in environments that appear to be uniformly unhealthy, there are usually choices if you really look and think creatively. At the corner store on the drive home from the beach, say, amid the neon-colored chips and soda, there's trail mix in the snacks section, yogurt in the refrigerator, and a basket of slightly bruised apples on the counter. Are those things perfect? No. But they're a lot better than the alternatives.

You now know how to take care of yourself. You know that means behaving in such a way that you meet your true needs instead of your immediate desires, cravings, and reactions. We'll all continue to be barraged by the presence of unhealthy foods and the constant messages, overt and subtle, that we're not good enough, that we need to be better— usually with the help of a product someone is selling, be it diet soda, a gym membership, a bikini, or a new car. That's a big part of why simply figuring out what's really going on, in our environments and within us, requires the process you've learned here, starting with slowing down and tuning in to yourself with curiosity and compassion.

And you know now that the more you care about yourself, the more you start expecting from your food: *Is this food worthy of me? Is the reason I'm eating, and the way I'm eating, worthy? Do my choices align with my values and support my health?* With practice and intention, you can move toward a place when the answer to those questions—not all of the time, but most of the time—is a resounding yes.

Acknowledgments

The authors would like to thank Duke Integrative Medicine for its support in bringing this project to life—in particular early cheerleaders Tracy Gaudet, M.D., and Isabel Geffner, who led the charge in bringing our work to a wider audience. Sincere thanks also to executive director Adam Perlman, M.D.; marketing director Eric T. Reese, M.B.A.; director of professional and public programs Linda Smith, PA-C, MS; and nutritionists Monica Gulisano, R.D., L.D.N., and Joanne Gardner, M.S., R.D.N., L.D.N.

We are deeply grateful to editor Shannon Welch at Scribner, who shaped *The Mindful Diet* so skillfully, and to Whitney Frick, the book's early champion. Thanks also to copy editor Lisa Wolff and production editor Mia Crowley.

Beth Reardon

I'd like to express sincere thanks to my brilliant coauthor Ruth, whose work in the area of mindfulness has been life-changing for so many people; to Tania Hannan, our writer, for her perseverance and commitment to translating the art and science of what we do at Duke Integrative Medicine; to Isabel Geffner, who helped me hone my sagas into sound bites; and to Doe Coover, our agent, for her never-ending support of our work and her words of wisdom.

Among the early inspirations for my work—and this book—were

my grandmother, Ann Torpey, whose Sunday dinners taught me life's sweetest lessons in "sufficiency" and whose very existence was an homage to selfless acts of kindness; Mary Feeney, the beloved babysitter who spent summers with us in Toms River and shared a recipe for the ages that came to define life's "whoopie-pie moments"; and the distinguished T. Collin Campbell, Ph.D., professor at Cornell, whose courses in Nutritional Biochemistry laid the foundation for my practice of integrative and functional nutrition at Duke.

Among the more recent inspirations, my many amazing colleagues at Duke IM, including Tracy Gaudet, M.D., our fearless leader, for having the courage to step into the space of integrative health care and for trusting us all to carry the torch for her vision, and Jeff Brantley, M.D., whose every word was a teaching moment, and whose contributions to Duke IM are immeasurable. I was inspired daily—and learned so much from—the gifted group of practitioners I had the privilege of working alongside: Louise Goldstein, R.N., nurse coordinator extraordinaire, who sailed us through exciting and stormy times with such grace, and who is the art and the heart of what we do; Janet Shaffer, L.Ac., the "needler's needler," who could take clients from 0–60 in one visit; Shelley Wroth, M.D., a Renaissance physician who could wear many hats (and look great in them); Eve Lausier, M.D., aka Mother Eve, whose beautiful singing was like a rheostat that brought us back to what mattered most and who taught me so much as I held on to her every word of dictation; Kim Turk, a skilled and gifted massage therapist who helped heal people in more ways than there are colors of kinesio tape; Sam Moon, M.D., my functional medicine sage; Michelle Bailey, M.D., and Susan Blackford, M.D., both gifts to their patients; Kelly Cross, L.M.T., massage therapist and accomplished artist; Jeanne van Gemert, L.M.B.T., L.P.C., who helps us make sense of ourselves with the help of unicorns, princes, and princesses, and who taught me how to breathe; and Carol Krucoff, E-RYT, internationally renowned teacher's teacher who gently heals our clients through purposeful movement.

Thanks also to Linda Smith, Director of Programs, who invited me into the world of Integrative Health Coaching, which forever changed how I practice (who knew you could teach so much in that space of listening?); to the entire program staff that made us look good; to health coaches Linda Duda, Julie Kosey, Jessica Wakefield, Cathy Parham, Andrea Shaw, and Kerry Little; and to extraordinary psychologists Janna Fikkan, Ph.D., my colead in the trenches who forgave me my poor translation of German, Jenn Davis, M.S., my other compassionate (and fashion-forward!) colead, and Jeff Greeson, Ph.D. Immense thanks to Cate Smith, soul sister and executive chef, who taught us all how to nourish our souls and feed our bodies with grace and gratitude; to Melva Strait Mary and La Wanna Bochert, who took such good care of all of us and our clients; and to Monica Gulisano, R.D., L.D.N., with whom I trust the mission for our patients.

Finally, to my husband, Dave, and daughters Meaghan, Delaney, and Calleigh: you are my life's whoopie-pie moments.

Ruth Quillian Wolever

I have so many people to thank who have knowingly or unknowingly directed my path: to Jim Spira, Ph.D., and Marty Sullivan, M.D., who introduced me to mindfulness and Claudia Plaisted Fernandez, Ph.D., who introduced me to conscious eating; to Jean Kristeller, Ph.D., who launched my study of mindful eating by inviting my partnership on her NIH-funded studies, and who continues to welcome my collaboration and challenge my thinking; to Sasha Loring, M.S., M.Ed., whose work and consistent support have guided and encouraged my efforts; to Jeff Brantley, M.D., who built the infrastructure to support my growth and that of many others in this practice; and to Jennifer Davis, M.S., who has continued to deepen my learning across the past two decades.

Many very special postdocs and colleagues have helped evaluate and refine this particular body of work. Among these are Janna Fikkan, Ph.D.; Jeff Greeson, Ph.D.; Jennifer Webb, Ph.D.; Julie Kosey, M.S.; Jessica Wakefield, M.A.; Barbara Culbertson, M.S.; and the Penn team including Larry Ladden, Ph.D.; Mara Wai, M.S.; and Michael Baime, M.D. Michael, in particular, helped me understand the application of mindfulness to behavior change in a much deeper way. I also deeply thank Karen Caldwell, Ph.D., and Kathy Buarotti for their generosity and incredible support; Michael Yapko, Ph.D., and his Chapel Hill team for encouraging constant discernment and laughter; and Tracy Gaudet, M.D., whose amazing ability to create reality from a compelling vision has steadily moved the entire field of integrative medicine forward for the past twenty years. I was honored to work by her side for ten of those years, and it was her vision to see this book in print.

Thanks to my dear family for sharing all that love and cookie dough (especially Frannie Joe), Mary Giannantonio for helping me to look more closely at myself, and all of Bug's team for clearing time for me to do this work. I am forever moved by the incredible acceptance and love of my husband, Mark, who consistently leads me to be a better person in my mindful and even my mindless moments. Thanks to Doe Coover, our agent, for her unflappable clarity and persistence; to my coauthor Beth Reardon, M.S., for her deep knowledge, creative spirit, and unbridled enthusiasm; and to Tania Hannan, whose unending patience and remarkable gift with words allowed us to make our knowledge and experience accessible to people in a way not otherwise possible. Finally, thanks to Kelley McCabe, M.B.A., who has been skillfully integrating the worlds of mindfulness and technology to disseminate this work through emindful.com.

Tania Hannan

To the brilliant, kind, and inspiring Beth Reardon and Ruth Quillian Wolever, I learned so much from you both—knowledge and wisdom—that I will carry with me; thank you. Sincere thanks also to Doe Coover and Isabel Geffner, for all the support, and to editors Shannon Welch and Whitney Frick, for your insights and guidance.

I am grateful to my extended family—Hannan, Tefft, Phillips, Williams, and McCleary clans—for the love, support, and patience during the writing process. Profound thanks also to my beloved family of friends—old and new, near and far—for our talks and walks, for your compassion, humor, and cheerleading. I'm grateful for having had two amazing teachers whose instruction, encouragement, and generosity of spirit have stayed with me and shaped my path: my high school English teacher Richard P. Russo and herbalist Rosemary Gladstar. To Elizabeth Barker, Kate Hanley, and Celina Ottaway, thank you. And to the staffs of Joe Van Gogh and Bean Traders, in Durham, N.C., where much of the first draft was written, thank you for the fuel and the friendliness.

Above all, I am grateful beyond words for my wife, Elizabeth Phillips, for things too numerous to mention, including having my back and holding my heart at all times.

Notes

Introduction

3   *Research shows that while:* T. Mann, A. J. Tomiyama, E. Westling, A. M. Lew, B. Samuels, and J. Chatman, "Medicare's Search for Effective Obesity Treatments: Diets Are Not the Answer," *American Psychologist* 62 (April 2007): 220-33, http://www.ncbi.nlm.nih.gov/pubmed/17469900; University of California—Los Angeles, "Dieting Does Not Work, Researchers Report," *ScienceDaily,* April 5, 2007, accessed February 11, 2014, www.sciencedaily.com/releases/2007/04/070404162428.htm.

Chapter 1: Why We Overeat

14   *Research shows that when:* Rose Oldham-Cooper et al., "Playing a Computer Game During Lunch Affects Fullness, Memory for Lunch, and Later Snack Intake," *American Journal of Clinical Nutrition* 93 (February 2011): 308–313, doi:10.3945/ajcn.110.004580.

17   *A Cornell University study compared:* B. Wansink, J. E. Painter, and Y. K. Lee, "The Office Candy Dish: Proximity's Influence on Estimated and Actual Consumption," *International Journal of Obesity* 30 (January 2006): 871–875, doi: 10.1038/sj.ijo.0803217; E. H. Castellanos, E. Charboneau, M. S. Dietrich, S. Park, B. P. Bradley, K. Mogg, and R. L. Cowan, "Obese Adults Have Visual Attention Bias for Food Cue Images: Evidence for Altered Reward System Function," *International Journal of Obesity* 33 (September 2009): 1063–73, doi:10.1038/ijo.2009.138.

17   *By some estimates, processed foods:* Kai Rissdal, *Processed Foods Make Up 70 Percent of the U.S. Diet,* podcast audio, March 12, 2013, http://www.marketplace.org/topics/life/big-book/processed-foods-make-70-percent-us-diet; Marion Nestle, "How Ultra-Processed Foods Are Killing Us," *The Atlantic,* November 4, 2010, http://www.theatlantic.com/health/archive/2010/11/how-ultra-processed-foods-are-killing-us/65614/; Carmen Piernas and Barry M. Popkin, "Snacking Increased among U.S. Adults Between 1977 and 2006," *Journal of Nutrition* 140 (February 2010): 325–332, doi: 10.3945/jn.109.112763; Hannah Fairfield, "Factory Food," *New York Times,* April 3, 2010, http://www.nytimes.com/2010/04/04/business/04metrics.html?_r=1; Sara N. Bleich, Y. Claire Wang, Youfa Wang, and Steven L. Gortmaker, "Increasing Consumption of Sugar-Sweetened Beverages among U.S. Adults: 1988–1994 to 1999–2004," *American Journal of Clinical Nutrition* 89 (January 2009): 372–81, doi:10.3945/ajcn.2008.26883.

18 *food companies create products:* Michael Moss, "The Extraordinary Power of Addictive Junk Food," *New York Times,* February 20, 2013, http://www.nytimes.com/2013 /02/24/magazine/the-extraordinary-science-of-junk-food.html?pagewanted=all& _r=0.

18 *One survey found that:* Lam Thuy Vo, "What America Spends on Groceries," *Planet Money* (blog), June 8, 2012, http://www.npr.org/blogs/money/2012/06/08 /154568945/what-america-spends-on-groceries.

18 *An article published:* Garry Welch, "Spending in the U.S. on Advertising for Fast Foods, Sodas, and Automobiles: Food for Thought Regarding the Type 2 Diabetes Epidemic," *Diabetes Care* 26 (February 2003) doi: 10.2337/diacare.26.2.546.

Chapter 2: What's on Your Plate?

28 *53 percent of overweight people:* Rebecca M. Puhl and Chelsea A. Heuer, "Public Opinion About Laws to Prohibit Weight Discrimination in the United States," *Obesity* 19 (January 2011): 74–82, doi:10.1038/oby.2010.126.

39 *Getting in touch with your values:* Kelly H. Webber, Deborah F. Tate, Dianne S. Ward, and J. Michael Bowling, "Motivation and Its Relationship to Adherence to Self-monitoring and Weight Loss in a 16-week Internet Behavioral Weight Loss Intervention," *Journal of Nutrition Education and Behavior* 42 (May-June 2010): 161– 67, doi:10.1016/j.jneb.2009.03.001; K. M. Flegal, M. D. Carroll, C. L. Ogden, and L. R. Curtin, "Prevalence and Trends in Obesity Among US Adults, 1999–2008," *Journal of the American Medical Association* 303 (January 2010: 235, doi:10.1001 /jama.2009.2014.

39 *Knowing Your Core Values:* The values exercise was adapted from the Personal Values Card Sort by W. R. Miller, J. C'de Baca, D. B. Matthews, and P. L. Wilbourne, University of New Mexico, 2001.

Chapter 3: Getting Off the Roller Coaster

43 *With nearly 70 percent of Americans:* "Obesity and Overweight," *Centers for Disease Control and Prevention,* last modified November 21, 2013. http://www.cdc.gov /nchs/fastats/overwt.htm; "100 Million Dieters, $20 Billion: The Weight-Loss Industry by the Numbers," *ABC News,* May 8, 2012, http://abcnews.go.com/Health /100-million-dieters-20-billion-weight-loss-industry/story?id=16297197; "Weight Loss Market in U.S. Up 1.7% to $61 Billion," *PR Web,* April 16, 2013, http://www .prweb.com/releases/2013/4/prweb10629316.htm.

43 *Many people who diet:* Stuart Wolpert, "Dieting Does Not Work, UCLA Researchers Report," *UCLA Newsroom,* April 3, 2007, http://www.newsroom.ucla.edu/portal /ucla/Dieting-Does-Not-Work-UCLA-Researchers-7832.aspx?RelNum=7832; James W. Anderson, Elizabeth C. Konz, Robert C. Frederich, and Constance L. Wood, "Long-Term Weight-Loss Maintenance: A Meta-Analysis of U.S. Studies," *American Journal of Clinical Nutrition* 74 (November 2001): 579–584, http://ajcn.nutrition .org/content/74/5/579.long; University of Melbourne, "Obese People Regain Weight After Dieting Due to Hormones, Australian Study Finds," *ScienceDaily,* October 31, 2011, www.sciencedaily.com/releases/2011/10/111028142504.htm; Christina Garcia Ulen, Mary Margaret Huizinga, MD, MPH, Bettina Beech, DrPH, and Tom A.

Elasy, MD, MPH, "Weight Gain Prevention," *Clinical Diabetes* 26 (July 2008): 100–13, doi:10.2337/diaclin.26.3.100.

49 *Health psychologists refer:* Susan Curry, Alan G. Marlatt, and Judith R. Gordon, "Abstinence Violation Effect: Validation of an Attributional Construct with Smoking Cessation," *Journal of Consulting and Clinical Psychology* 55 (April 1987): 145–59, doi:10.1037/0022-006X.55.2.145.

54 *According to the Centers for Disease Control:* "Exercise or Physical Activity," *Centers for Disease Control and Prevention,* last modified February 28, 2014, http://www .cdc.gov/nchs/fastats/exercise.htm.

56 *But substituting synthetic ingredients:* "FDA Should Reconsider Aspartame Cancer Risk, Say Experts," *Center for Science in the Public Interest,* June 25, 2007, https:// www.cspinet.org/new/200706251.html, "It's Sweet . . . But Is It Safe?" *Center for Science in the Public Interest,* December 31, 2013, http://www.cspinet.org/new /201312311.html.

57 *A recent population study also showed:* Guy Fagherazzi, Alice Vilier, Daniela Saes Sartorelli, Martin Lajous, Beverley Balkau, and Françoise Clavel-Chapelon, "Consumption of Artificially and Sugar-Sweetened Beverages and Incident Type 2 Diabetes in the E3N-EPIC Cohort," *American Journal of Clinical Nutrition* 97 (January 2013): 517–23, doi:10.3945/ajcn.112.050997; " 'Diet' drinks associated with increased risk of Type II diabetes," *Inserm,* February 7, 2013, http://english.inserm.fr /press-area/diet-drinks-associated-with-increased-risk-of-type-ii-diabetes; Charlene Leno, "Is Diet Soda Linked to Heart, Stroke Risk?" *WebMD Stroke Health Center,* last modified 2011, http://www.webmd.com/stroke/news/20110209/is-diet -soda-linked-to-heart-stroke-risk.

60 *we often coach patients to create:* Goal-setting exercises adapted from programs used by the Duke Diet and Fitness Center.

Chapter 4: The Practice of Change

67 *At the University of Massachusetts Medical Center:* University of Massachusetts Medical School, "Major Research Studies and Findings," *Center for Mindfulness in Medicine, Health Care and Society,* http://www.umassmed.edu/Content.aspx?id=42426.

71 *In one study of MBSR participants:* F. Zeidan, K. T. Martucci, R. A. Kraft, J. G. McHaffie, and R. C. Coghill, "Neural Correlates of Mindfulness Meditation-Related Anxiety Relief," *Social Cognitive and Affective Neuroscience* (June 2013), doi:10.1093 /scan/nst041; Sara W. Lazar, "Meditation and Neuroplasticity," *International Congress on Mindfulness,* http://www.achtsamkeitskongress.de/index.php?id=635&L=1.

76 *In several NIH-funded clinical trials:* From the pilot trial: J. L. Kristeller and B. C. Hallet (1999). An exploratory study of meditation-based intervention for binge eating disorder. *Journal of Health Psychology* 4 (3), 357–63; from NIH grant R21 AT000416 to PI Kristeller at ISU (Site PI Wolever at Duke): J. L. Kristeller, R. A. Baer, and R. E. Quillian-Wolever (2006). Mindfulness-Based approaches to eating disorders. In R. A. Baer (ed.), *Mindfulness-Based Treatment Approaches: Clinician's Guide to Evidence Base and Applications* (pp. 75–91). New York: Elsevier; J. L. Kristeller and R. Q. Wolever (2011). Mindfulness-Based Eating Awareness Training for Treating Binge Eating Disorder: The conceptual foundation. *Eating Disorders: The Journal of Treatment and Prevention* 19(1), 49–61; J. L. Kristeller, R. Q. Wolever, and

V. Sheets (2013). Mindfulness-Based Eating Awareness Treatment (MB-EAT) for Binge Eating Disorder: A Randomized Clinical Trial. *Mindfulness*, doi: 10.1007/ s12671-012-0179-1; J. L. Kristeller and R. Q. Wolever (2013). Mindfulness-Based Eating Awareness Training for Treating Binge Eating Disorder: The conceptual foundation. In L. M. DeSole (ed.), *Eating Disorders and Mindfulness: Exploring Alternative Approaches to Treatment*. New York: Routledge. From NIH linked grants U01 AT004159 to PI Wolever at Duke and U01 AT004158 to PI Baime at Penn: R. Q. Wolever and J. L. Best (2009). Mindfulness-Based approaches to eating disorders. In F. Didonna (ed.), *Clinical Handbook of Mindfulness* (pp. 259–287). New York: Springer; K. Caldwell, M. Baime, and R. Q. Wolever (2012). Mindfulness-Based Approaches to Obesity and Weight Loss Maintenance. *Journal of Mental Health Counseling* 34(3), 269–82; K. L. Caldwell, J. Grey, and R. Q. Wolever (2013). The process of patient empowerment in integrative health coaching: how does it happen? *Global Advances in Health and Medicine*, 2(3), 48–57. From NIH grant U01 AT002550 to PI Kristeller at ISU (Co-PI Wolever and team at Duke co-developed treatment and operations manuals 2006–2007 only, while Kristeller and team did the entire data collection and analysis for this trial): J. L. Kristeller and R. Q. Wolever (2014). Mindfulness-Based Eating Awareness Training: Treatment of Overeating and Obesity. In R. A. Baer (ed.), *Mindfulness-Based Treatment Approaches: Clinician's Guide to Evidence Base and Applications*. Burlington, MA: Academic Press, 119– 39; J. L. Kristeller and R. Q. Wolever (under contract). *Mindfulness-Based Eating Awareness Training (MB-EAT): Clinician's Manual*. New York: Guildford. *Metabolic Syndrome and Weight Loss Study: A Randomized Controlled Trial of Behavioral Interventions* is an industry trial sponsored by emindful.com and Aetna (2010–2014), with completed data collection and preliminary analyses. Follow-up analyses and manuscripts are currently in preparation at the time this book went to press.

86 *A study of eighty-four women:* Claire E. Adams and Mark R. Leary, "Promoting Self-Compassionate Attitudes Toward Eating Among Restrictive and Guilty Eaters," *Journal of Social and Clinical Psychology* 26, no. 10 (2007): 1120–44, doi:10.1521 /jscp.2007.26.10.1120.

95 *Mindfulness tool: Body Scan:* Body Scan adapted from Edward A. Charlesworth and Ronald G. Nathan, *Stress Management: A Comprehensive Guide to Wellness* (New York: Ballantine, 2004); Jon Kabat-Zinn, *Full Catastrophe Living* (New York: Bantam, 2013).

Chapter 5: The Goldilocks Principle

105 *The Science of Appetite:* David E. Cummings and Joost Overduin, "Gastrointestinal Regulation of Food Intake," *Journal of Clinical Investigation* 117 (January 2007): 13–23, doi: 10.1172/JCI30227; A. Kong, M. L. Neuhouser, L. Xiao, C. M. Ulrich, A. McTiernan, and K. E. Foster-Schubert, "Higher Habitual Intake of Dietary Fat and Carbohydrates Are Associated with Lower Leptin and Higher Ghrelin Concentrations in Overweight and Obese Postmenopausal Women with Elevated Insulin Levels," *Nutrition Research* 29 (November 2009): 768–76, doi:10.1016/j .nutres.2009.10.013; Neil A. Schwarz, B. Rhett Rigby, Paul La Bounty, Brian Shelmadine, and Rodney G. Bowden, "A Review of Weight Control Strategies and Their Effects on the Regulation of Hormonal Balance," *Journal of Nutrition and Metabolism*

2011 (July 2011), doi:10.1155/2011/237932; A. Lindqvist, C. D. de la Cour, A. Steg-mark, R. Håkanson, and C. Erlanson-Albertsson, "Overeating of Palatable Food Is Associated with Blunted Leptin and Ghrelin Responses," *Regulatory Peptides* 130 (September 2005): 123–32, doi:10.1016/j.regpep.2005.05.002; Martin G. Myers, Jr., Rudolph L. Leibel, Randy J. Seeley, and Michael W. Schwartz, "Obesity and Leptin Resistance: Distinguishing Cause from Effect," *Trends in Endocrinology & Metabolism* 21 (September 2010): 643–51, doi:10.1016/j.tem.2010.08.002; H. Fink, A. Rex, M. Voits, and J. P. Voigt, "Major Biological Actions of CCK—A Critical Evaluation of Research Findings," *Experimental Brain Research* 123 (October 1998): 77–83, doi:10.1007/s002210050546.

113 *Researchers at Australia's:* S. L. Leong, C. Madden, A. Gray, D. Waters, and C. Hor-wath, "Faster Self-Reported Speed of Eating Is Related to Higher Body Mass Index in a Nationwide Survey of Middle-Aged Women," *Journal of the American Dietetic Association* 111 (August 2011): 1192–97, doi:10.1016/j.jada.2011.05.012.

114 *But shifting to* enough: BMJ-British Medical Journal, "Eating Quickly and Until Full Triples Risk of Being Overweight," *ScienceDaily,* October 22, 2008, www.science daily.com/releases/2008/10/081021210307.htm.

121 *The idea that the mind and body are separate:* "Mind-Body Dualism," *Encyclopaedia Britannica,* http://www.britannica.com/EBchecked/topic/383566/mind-body -dualism.

Chapter 6: The Pleasure Principle

124 *Researchers at Yale University:* A. J. Crum, W. R. Corbin, K. D. Brownell, and P. Sa-lovey, "Mind Over Milkshakes: Mindsets, Not Just Nutrients, Determine Ghrelin Response," *Health Psychology Advance* (May 16, 2011): doi: 10.1037/a0023467.

129 *Research suggests that satiety:* Devina Wadhera, E. D. Capaldi, and L. Wilkie, "Mul-tiple Pieces of Food Are More Rewarding Than an Equicaloric Single Piece of Food in Both Animals and Humans" (presentation, Annual Meeting of the Society for the Study of Ingestive Behavior, Zurich, Switzerland, July 10–14, 2012).

129 *Research and our clinical experience:* H. A. Raynor and L. H. Epstein, "Dietary Variety, Energy Regulation, and Obesity," *Psychological Bulletin* 127 (May 2001): 325–41, http://www.ncbi.nlm.nih.gov/pubmed/11393299.

129 *When complex flavors are involved:* L. B. Sørensen, P. Møller, A. Flint, M. Martens, and A. Raben, "Effect of Sensory Perception of Foods on Appetite and Food In-take: A Review of Studies on Humans," *International Journal of Obesity and Related Metabolic Disorders* 27 (October 2003): 1152–66, http://www.ncbi.nlm.nih.gov /pubmed/14513063; M. Romer, J. Lerhner, V. Van Wymbelbeke, T. Jiang, L. Deecke, and L. Brondel, "Does Modification of Olfacto-Gustatory Stimulation Diminish Sensory-Specific Satiety in Humans?" *Physiology & Behavior* 87 (March 2006): 469–77, http://www.ncbi.nlm.nih.gov/pubmed/16458336.

130 *Some studies suggest:* Amanda B. Maliphol, Deborah J. Garth, and Kathryn F. Medler, "Diet-Induced Obesity Reduces the Responsiveness of the Peripheral Taste Re-ceptor Cells," *PLoS ONE 8* (November 2013): doi: 10.1371/journal.pone.0079403; Society for the Study of Ingestive Behavior, "Obesity Is Associated with Reduced Sensitivity to Fat," *ScienceDaily,* July 19, 2010, www.sciencedaily.com/releases/2010 /07/100713011045.htm; Penn State, "Route to Obesity Passes Through Tongue,"

ScienceDaily, November 28, 2008, http://www.sciencedaily.com/releases/2008/11
/081126133409.htm.

130 *One recent study showed:* Johanna Overberg, Thomas Hummel, Heiko Krude, and
Susanna Wiegand, "Differences in Taste Sensitivity Between Obese and Non-Obese
Children and Adolescents," *Archives of Disease in Childhood* 97 (December 2012):
1048–1052, doi: 10.1136/archdischild-2011-301189.

130 *Research shows that compared:* Siew Ling Tey, Rachel C. Brown, Andrew R. Gray,
Alexandra W. Chishold, and Conor M. Delahunty, "Long-term Consumption of
High Energy-Dense Snack Foods on Sensory-Specific Satiety and Intake," *American Journal of Clinical Nutrition* 95 (May 2012): 1038–1047, doi: 10.3945/ajcn.111
.030882.

131 *Food companies are well versed:* A. N. Gearhardt, C. Davis, R. Kuschner, and
K. D. Brownell, "The Addiction Potential of Hyperpalatable Foods," *Current Drug
Abuse Reviews* 4 (September 2011): 140–45, http://www.ncbi.nlm.nih.gov/pubmed
/21999688.

131 *Food companies have taken the flavors:* Magalie Lenoir, Fuschia Serre, Lauriane
Cantin, and Serge H. Ahmed, "Intense Sweetness Surpasses Cocaine Reward," *PLoS
ONE* 2 (August 2007): e698, doi: 10.1371/journal.pone.0698.

131 *There's evidence that on a chemical level:* George A. Bray, Samara Joy Nielsen, and
Barry M. Popkin, "Consumption of High-Fructose Corn Syrup in Beverages May
Play a Role in the Epidemic of Obesity," *American Journal of Clinical Nutrition* 79
(April 2004): 537–43, www.ajcn.org/content/79/4/537.full.

131 *In one recent study, when people:* Nathan Gray, "Low calorie sweetener may not increase satiety, suggests study," FoodNavigator.com, January 26, 2011, http://www
.foodnavigator.com/Science-Nutrition/Low-calorie-sweetener-may-not-increase
-satiety-suggests-study.

132 *You can recalibrate your taste satiety:* Richard D. Mattes and Barry M. Popkin, "Non-nutritive sweetener consumption in humans: effects on appetite and food intake
and their putative mechanisms," *International Journal of Obesity Related Metabolic
Disorders* 67 (January 1999): 80–86, http://ajcn.nutrition.org/content/89/1/1.full;
A. Kokkinos, C. W. le Roux, K. Alexiadou, N. Tentolouris, R. P. Vincent, D. Kyriaki,
D. Perrea, M. A. Ghatei, S. R. Bloom, and N. Katsilambros, "Eating Slowly Increases the Postprandial Response of the Anorexigenic Gut Hormones, Peptide YY
and Glucagon-Like Peptide-1," *Journal of Clinical Endocrinology and Metabolism*
95 (January 2010): 333–37,doi:10.1210/jc.2009-1018; Nicolien Zijlstra, René A.
de Wijk, Monica Mars, Annette Stafleu, and Cees de Graaf, "Effect of Bite Size and
Oral Processing Time of a Semisolid Food on Satiation," *American Journal of Clinical Nutrition* 90 (August 2009): 269–75. doi: 10.3945/ajcn.2009.27694.

133 *Some 18 percent of our calories:* USDA, "Beverage Choices of U.S. Adults, NHANES
Survey 2007–2008," dietary data brief (August 2011), https://www.ars.usda.gov
/SP2UserFiles/Place/12355000/pdf/DBrief/6_beverage_choices_adults_0708.pdf.

133 *In fact, a recent Johns Hopkins study:* Johns Hopkins Bloomberg School of Public Health, "Beverage Consumption a Bigger Factor in Weight," news release,
April 2, 2009, http://www.jhsph.edu/news/news-releases/2009/caballero_beverage
_consumption.html.

133 *If you think you can have the best:* P. A. Smeets, P. Weijzen, C. de Graaf, and
M. A. Viergever, "Consumption of Caloric and Non-Caloric Versions of a Soft

Drink Differentially Affects Brain Activation During Tasting," *Neuroimage* 54 (January 2011): 1367–74, doi: 10.1016/j.neuroimage.2010.08.054.

Chapter 7: A Cure for Emotional Eating

145 *People who are overweight:* S. Pinaquy, H. Chabrol, C. Simon, J. P. Louvet, and P. Barbe, "Emotional Eating, Alexithymia, and Binge-Eating Disorder in Obese Women," *Obesity Research* 11 (February 2003): 195–201, http://www.ncbi.nlm.nih.gov/pubmed/12582214.

154 *One sign of our relaxation deficiency:* American Psychological Association, "Understanding Chronic Stress," http://www.apa.org/helpcenter/understanding-chronic-stress.aspx (n.d.).

155 *One study, for instance, showed:* Jennifer Daubenmier, Jean Kristeller, Frederick M. Hecht, et al., "Mindfulness Intervention for Stress Eating to Reduce Cortisol and Abdominal Fat among Overweight and Obese Women: An Exploratory Randomized Controlled Study," *Journal of Obesity*, vol. 2011 (2011), Article ID 651936, doi:10.1155/2011/651936.

157 *One of these is a well-researched neurotransmitter:* Colette Bouchez, "Serotonin: 9 Questions and Answers," WebMD.com Depression Health Center, http://www.webmd.com/depression/features/serotonin.

158 *Studies have shown that carbohydrates:* Paul M. Johnson and Paul J. Kenny, "Addiction-like Reward Dysfunction and Compulsive Eating in Obese Rats: Role for Dopamine D2 Receptors," *Nature Neuroscience* 13 (2010): 635–41, doi: 10.1038/nn.2519.

158 *In a double-blind, placebo-controlled study:* J. D. Lane, C. F. Pieper, B. G. Phillips-Bute, J. E. Bryant, and C. M. Kuhn, "Caffeine Affects Cardiovascular and Neuroendocrine Activation at Work and Home," *Psychosomatic Medicine* 64 (2002): 595–603, doi: 10.1097/01.PSY.0000021946.90613.DB; Duke Medicine News and Communications, "Caffeine's Effects Are Long-Lasting and Compound Stress," Duke University's health library, July 26, 2002, http://www.dukehealth.org/health_library/news/5687.

159 *One recent study of women:* A. Janet Tomiyama, Mary F. Dallman, and Elissa S. Epel, "Comfort Food Is Comforting to Those Most Stressed: Evidence of the Chronic Stress Response Network in High Stress Women," *Psychoneuroendocrinology* 36 (November 2011): 1513–1519, http://www.sciencedirect.com/science/article/pii/S0306453011001296; Jeffrey Norris, "Comfort Food May Be 'Self-Medication' for Stress, Dialing Down Stress Response," University of California San Francisco (December 7, 2011), http://www.ucsf.edu/news/2011/12/11089/comfort-food-may-be-self-medication-stress-dialing-down-stress-response.

160 *Knowing the biology of mood and food:* Simon N. Young, "How to Increase Serotonin in the Human Brain Without Drugs," *Journal of Psychiatry and Neuroscience* 32 (November 2007): 394–99, http://www.ncbi.nlm.nih.gov/pmc/articles/PMC2077351/.

Chapter 8: A Body to Love

165 *How we view our bodies:* E. V. Carraça, M. N. Silva, D. Markland, P. N. Vieira, C. S. Minderico, L. B. Sardinha, P. and J. Teixeira, "Body Image Change and Improved Eating Self-Regulation in a Weight Management Intervention in Women," *The International Journal of Behavioral Nutrition and Physical Activity* 8 (July 18, 2011): 75, doi: 10.1186/1479-5868-8-75.

171 *In one study, children as young:* Emma C. Spiel, Susan J. Paxton, and Zali Yager, "Weight Attitudes in 3- to 5-year-old Children: Age Differences and Cross-Sectional Predictors," *Body Image* 9 (September 2012): 524–27, http://www.sciencedirect.com /science/article/pii/S1740144512000927.

Chapter 9: Know Your Triggers

189 *Using a technique called chain analysis:* The chain analysis technique was developed for use in dialectical behavior therapy (DBT).

Chapter 10: The Four Pillars of Healthy Eating

208 *From a public-health perspective:* Centers for Disease Control and Prevention, "Chronic Diseases: The Power to Prevent, the Call to Control: At a Glance 2009," http://www.cdc.gov/chronicdisease/resources/publications/aag/chronic.htm; Loren Cordain, S. Boyd Eaton, Anthony Sebastian, Neil Mann, Staffan Lindeber, Bruce A. Watkins, James H. O'Keefe, and Janette Brand-Miller, "Origins and Evolution of the Western Diet: Health Implications for the 21st Century," *American Journal of Clinical Nutrition* 81 (February 2005): 341–54, http://ajcn.nutrition.org/content/81 /2/341.full.

209 *today Americans consume on average:* R. Bethene Ervin and Cynthia L. Ogden, "Consumption of Added Sugars Among U.S. Adults, 2005–2010," NHCS Data Brief 22 (May 2013), http://www.cdc.gov/nchs/data/databriefs/db122.htm.

209 *Less than 25 percent of adults:* CDC, "Chronic Diseases and Health Promotion" (August 2012), http://www.cdc.gov/chronicdisease/overview/index.htm.

210 *According to the USDA:* U.S. Department of Agriculture, U.S. Department of Health and Human Services, *Dietary Guidelines for Americans,* http://www.fns.usda.gov /sites/default/files/Chapter2.pdf.

214 *Trans fats, man-made fats found:* Harvard School of Public Health, "Shining the Spotlight on Trans Fats," http://www.hsph.harvard.edu/nutritionsource/transfats/#6.

217 *according to a recent report:* G. M. Reaven, "Insulin Resistance: The Link Between Obesity and Cardiovascular Disease," *Medical Clinics of North America* 95 (September 2011): 875–92, doi: 10.1016/j.mcna.2011.06.002.

218 *researchers have been investigating:* Rachael Z. Stolzenberg-Solomon, Barry I. Graubard, Suresh Chari, Paul Limburg, Philip R. Taylor, Jarmo Virtamo, and Demetrius Albanes, "Insulin, Glucose, Insulin Resistance, and Pancreatic Cancer in Male Smokers," *Journal of the American Medical Association* 294 (2005): 2872–78, doi:10.1001/jama.294.22.2872.

219 *A tool called the glycemic index:* Harvard Medical School, "Glycemic Index and Glycemic Load for 100+ Foods," Harvard University, Harvard Health Publications,

http://www.health.harvard.edu/newsweek/Glycemic_index_and_glycemic_load_for _100_foods.htm.

223 *Recognizing these risks, the FDA:* "Harkin Welcomes FDA Move to Remove 'Generally Recognized as Safe' Status for Trans Fats," news release from the U.S. Senate Committee on Health Education, Labor, and Pensions (November 7, 2013), http:// www.help.senate.gov/newsroom/press/release/?id=3bbe737e-5057-40d6-9f4b-f90 b72e9dd7b.

225 *Some studies even show that:* Johns Hopkins Medicine, "Nutrition and Colon Cancer: Eating to Fight and Prevent Colorectal Cancer," http://hopkinscoloncancercenter.org /CMS/CMS_Page.aspx?CurrentUDV=59&CMS_Page_ID=8345F49E-9814-467C -B7F3-A68FC4C6FE96.

225 *Recent studies have linked:* K. M. Tuohy, L. Conterno, M. Gasperotti, and R. Viola, "Up-regulating the Human Intestinal Microbiome Using Whole Plant Foods, Polyphenols, and/or Fiber," *Journal of Agriculture and Food Chemistry* 60 (September 12, 2012): 8776–82. doi: 10.1021/jf2053959.

227 *In a recent study published:* M. Karalus, M. Clark, K. A. Greaves, W. Thomas, Z. Vickers, M. Kuyama, and J. Slavin, "Fermentable Fibers Do Not Affect Satiety or Food Intake by Women Who Do Not Practice Restrained Eating," *Journal of the Academy of Nutrition and Dietetics* 112 (September 2012): 1356–62, doi: 10.1016 /j.jand.2012.05.022.

229 *For a report published in:* F. B. Hu, "Plant-based Foods and Prevention of Cardiovascular Disease: An Overview," *American Journal of Clinical Nutrition* 78 (September 2003): 544S–551S, https://www.ncbi.nlm.nih.gov/pubmed/12936948.

230 *And some research, including one study:* N. D. Barnard, A. R. Scialli, G. Turner-McGrievy, A. J. Lanou, and J. Glass, "The Effects of a Low-Fat, Plant-Based Dietary Intervention on Body Weight, Metabolism, and Insulin Sensitivity," *American Journal of Medicine* 118 (September 2005): 991–97, https://www.ncbi.nlm.nih .gov/pubmed/?term=2005+American+Journal+of+Medicine+plant-based+weight +loss.

230 *as well as the growth-hormone residue:* Samuel S. Epstein, "Hormones in U.S. Beef Linked to Increased Cancer Risk," Cancer Prevention Coalition press release (October 21, 2009), http://world-wire.com/news/0910210001.html; The American Cancer Society's information page on recombinant bovine growth hormone, http://www .cancer.org/cancer/cancercauses/othercarcinogens/athome/recombinant-bovine -growth-hormone.

230 *Plant-based protein can also provide:* Kristen S. Montgomery, "Soy Protein," *Journal of Perinatal Education* 12 (Summer 2003), 42–45, doi: 10.1624/105812403X106946.

233 *Animal research also demonstrates:* G. J. Mazza, "Anthocyanins and Heart Health," *Annali dell'Istituto Superiore Sanità* 43 (2007): 369–74, https://www.ncbi.nlm.nih .gov/pubmed/18209270; A. Basu, M. Rhone, and T. J. Lyons, "Berries: Emerging Impact on Cardiovascular Health," *Nutrition Reviews* 68 (March 2010): 168–77, doi: 10.1111/j.1753-4887.2010.00273.x; A. Cassidy, E. J. O'Reilly, C. Kay, L. Sampson, M. Franz, J. P. Forman, G. Curhan, and E. B. Rimm, "Habitual Intake of Flavonoid Subclasses and Incident Hypertension in Adults," *American Journal of Clinical Nutrition* 93 (February 2011): 338–47, doi: 10.3945/ajcn.110.006783; R. L. Prior, X. Wu, L. Gu, T. J. Hager, A. Hager, and L. R. Howard, "Whole Berries versus Berry Anthocyanins: Interactions with Dietary Fat Levels in the C57BL/6J Mouse Model

of Obesity," *Journal of Agriculture and Food Chemistry* 56 (February 2008): 647–53, doi: 10.1021/jf0719930.

234 *cruciferous vegetables:* Information on phytochemicals from the Linus Pauling Institute's Micronutrient Information Center, http://lpi.oregonstate.edu/infocenter /phytochemicals/i3c/.

235 *Animal research suggests:* USDA/Agricultural Research Service, "Compound in Turmeric Spice May Stall Spread of Fat Tissue," *ScienceDaily*, May 25, 2009, www .sciencedaily.com/releases/2009/05/090522181238.htm.

Chapter 11: How Much Food Do You Really Need?

243 *A supersized soft drink:* Aaron Edwards, "At 7-11, the Big Gulps Elude a Ban by the City," *New York Times*, June 6, 2012, http://www.nytimes.com/2012/06/07/nyregion /7-eleven-big-gulps-are-immune-from-proposed-new-york-city-ban.html.

244 *Consider how portion sizes have grown:* "The New Abnormal," Centers for Disease Control and Prevention, http://makinghealtheasier.org/newabnormal; "Portion Distortion: Serving Sizes Are Growing," Naval Medical Center San Diego, http:// www.med.navy.mil/sites/nmcsd/Patients/Pages/PortionDistortion-ServingSizesare Growing.aspx.

246 *In one study, for example:* B. J. Rolls, L. S. Roe, J. S. Meengs, and D. E. Wall, "Increasing the Portion Size of a Sandwich Increases Energy Intake," *Journal of the American Dietetic Association* 104 (March 2004): 367–72, https://www.ncbi.nlm.nih.gov /pubmed/14993858.

251 *We have a harder time judging portions:* Jenny H. Ledikew, Julia A. Ello-Martin, and Barbara J. Rolls, "Portion Sizes and the Obesity Epidemic," *Journal of Nutrition* 4 (April 2005): 905–909, http://jn.nutrition.org/content/135/4/905.long.

252 *Eating and drinking between meals:* K. J. Duffey and B. M. Popkin, "Energy Density, Portion Size, and Eating Occasions: Contributions to Increased Energy Intake in the United States, 1977–2006," *PLoS Medicine* 8 (June 28, 2011), doi:10.1371 /journal.pmed.1001050; "Snacking Constitutes 25 Percent of Calories Consumed in U.S.," Institute for Food Technologists, June 20, 2011, http://www.ift.org/newsroom /news-releases/2011/june/20/snacking-constitutes-25-percent-of-calories-consumed -in-us.aspx.

252 *Processed snack foods:* Jennifer L. Harris, Megan E. Weinberg, Marlene B. Schwartz, Craig Ross, Joshua Ostroff, and Kelly D. Brownell, "Rudd Report: Trends in Television Food Advertising," February 2010, http://www.yaleruddcenter.org/resources /upload/docs/what/reports/RuddReport_TVFoodAdvertising_2.10.pdf.

255 *Like other fast-burning carbs, sugary drinks:* D. P. DiMeglio and R. D. Mattes, "Liquid versus Solid Carbohydrate: Effects on Food Intake and Body Weight," *International Journal of Obesity Related Metabolic Disorders* 24 (June 2): 794–800, https://www .ncbi.nlm.nih.gov/pubmed/10878689.

255 *Artificially sweetened soft drinks:* Qing Yang, "Gain Weight by 'Going Diet?' Artificial Sweeteners and the Neurobiology of Sugar Cravings," *Yale Journal of Biology and Medicine* 83 (2) (June 2010): 101–108, http://www.ncbi.nlm.nih.gov/pmc /articles/PMC2892765/.

258 *However, a few recent studies suggest:* Megumi Hatori, Christopher Vollmers, Amir Zarrinpar, Luciano DiTacchio, Eric A. Bushong, Shubhroz Gill, Mathias Leblanc,

Amandine Chaix, Matthew Joens, James A. J. Fitzpatrick, Mark H. Ellisman, and Satchidananda Panda, "Time-Restricted Feeding without Reducing Caloric Intake Prevents Metabolic Diseases in Mice Fed a High-Fat Diet," *Cell Metabolism* (2012), doi: 10.1016/j.cmet.2012.04.019.

259 *Research shows that people who skip breakfast:* C. Horikawa, S. Kodama, Y. Yachi, Y. Heianza, R. Hirasawa, Y. Ibe, K. Saito, H. Shimano, N. Yamada, and H. Sone, "Skipping Breakfast and Prevalence of Overweight and Obesity in Asian and Pacific Regions: A Meta-Analysis," *Preventive Medicine* 53 (October 2011): 260–67, doi: 10.1016/j.ypmed.2011.08.030; Institute of Food Technologists, "Skipping Breakfast Can Lead to Unhealthy Habits All Day Long," *ScienceDaily*, June 29, 2012, www .sciencedaily.com/releases/2012/06/120629143045.htm; H. R. Wyatt, G. K. Grunwald, C. L. Mosca, M. L. Klem, R. R. Wing, and J. O. Hill, "Long-term Weight Loss and Breakfast in Subjects in the National Weight Control Registry," *Obesity Research* 10 (February 2002): 78–82, https://www.ncbi.nlm.nih.gov/pubmed/11836452.

Chapter 12: Reconnecting with Your Food

272 *Studies have consistently shown:* Valdimar Sigurdsson, Hugi Saevarsson, and Gordon Foxall, "Brand Placement and Consumer Choice: An In-Store Experiment," *Journal of Applied Behavior Analysis* 42 (Fall 2009): 741–45, doi: 10.1901/jaba.2009.42-741.

272 *As you've learned, HFCS appears:* Hillary Parker, "A Sweet Problem: Princeton Researchers Find that High-Fructose Corn Syrup Prompts Considerably More Weight Gain," *News at Princeton* (March 22, 2010), https://www.princeton.edu /main/news/archive/S26/91/22K07/.

298 *A regular practice of focusing on thankful feelings:* Robert Emmons, "Why Gratitude Is Good," The Greater Good Science Center, University of California, Berkeley, November 16, 2010, http://greatergood.berkeley.edu/article/item/why_gratitude_is _good/.

300 *In fact, 47 percent of all the money spent on food:* National Restaurant Association information page, "Facts at a Glance," http://www.restaurant.org/News-Research /Research/Facts-at-a-Glance.

300 *typical restaurant meals average:* M. J. Scourboutakos, Z. Semnani-Azad, and M. R. L'Abbe, "Restaurant Meals: Almost a Full Day's Worth of Calories, Fats, and Sodium," *Journal of the American Medical Association Internal Medicine*, 2013, 173(14): 1373–74, doi:10.1001/jamainternmed.2013.6159.

303 *Research has shown that people given alcohol:* S. J. Caton, L. Bate, and M. M. Hetherington, "Acute Effects of an Alcoholic Drink on Food Intake: Aperitif versus Co-Ingestion," *Physiological Behavior* 90 (2–3) (Feb 2007): 368–75, doi: 10.1016/j .physbeh.2006.09.028.

303 *Calorie Counts for Common Drinks:* National Institute on Alcohol Abuse and Alcoholism, "Rethinking Drinking," http://rethinkingdrinking.niaaa.nih.gov/Tools Resources/CalorieCalculator.asp.

Index